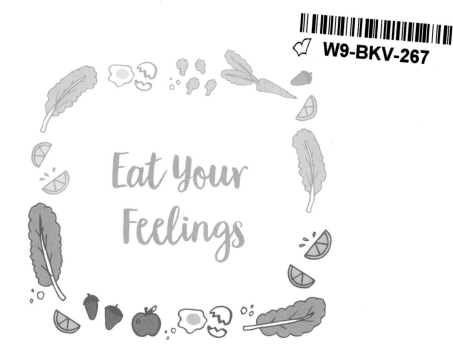

Eat Your Feelings

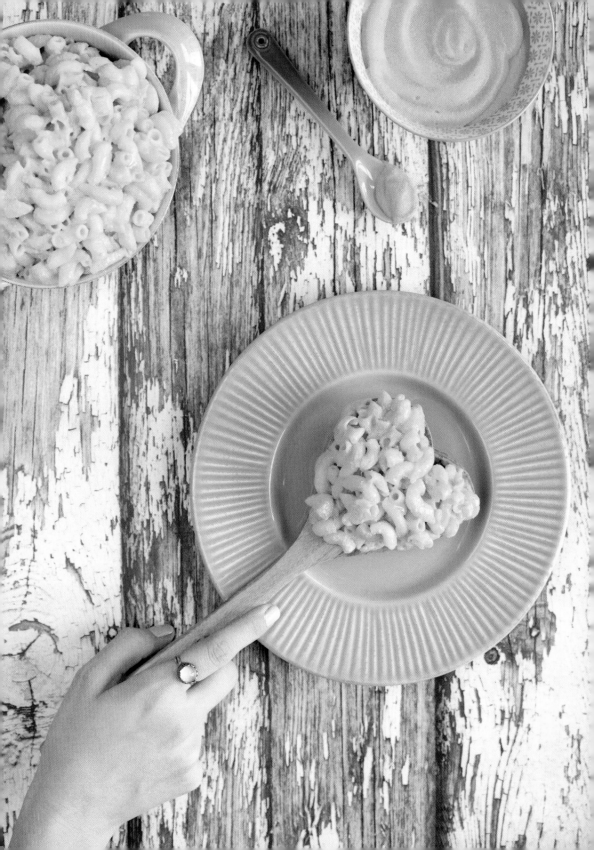

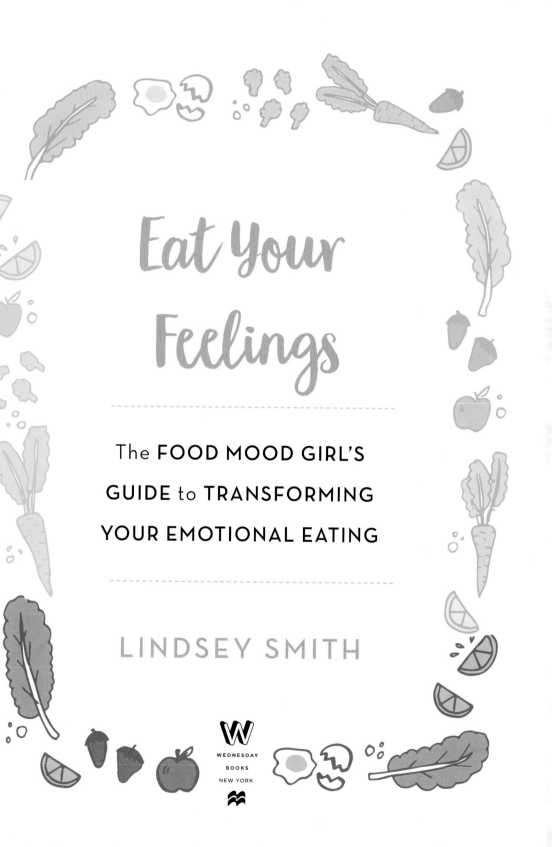

Eat Your Feelings

The **FOOD MOOD GIRL'S**
GUIDE to **TRANSFORMING**
YOUR EMOTIONAL EATING

LINDSEY SMITH

WEDNESDAY
BOOKS
NEW YORK

To my adorable pup, Winnie Cooper.
May your mood be ever improved from eating
all the scraps off the kitchen floor during the creation of this book.

www.stmartins.com

Book design by Susan Walsh
Photography by Sarah VanTassel
Illustrations by Kate Reingold
Food styling by Quelcy Kogel

The Library of Congress Cataloging-in-Publication Data is available upon request.

ISBN 978-1-250-13941-2 (trade paperback)
ISBN 978-1-250-13942-9 (ebook)

Our books may be purchased in bulk for promotional, educational, or business use. Please contact your local bookseller or the Macmillan Corporate and Premium Sales Department at 1-800-221-7945, extension 5442, or by email at MacmillanSpecialMarkets@macmillan.com.

First Edition: January 2018

10 9 8 7 6 5 4 3 2 1

Contents

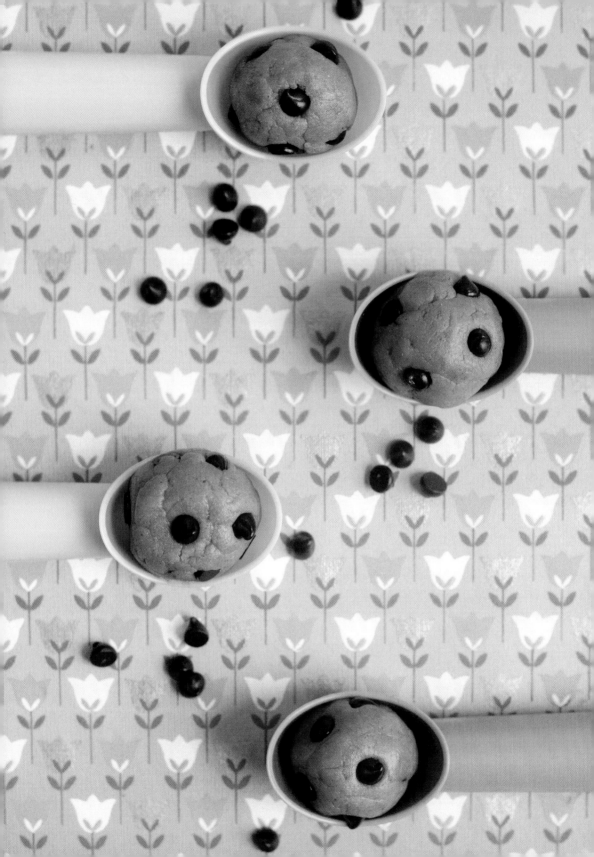

You are not alone.

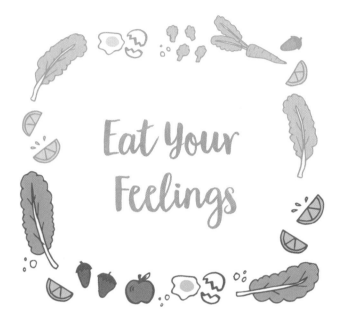

Eat Your Feelings

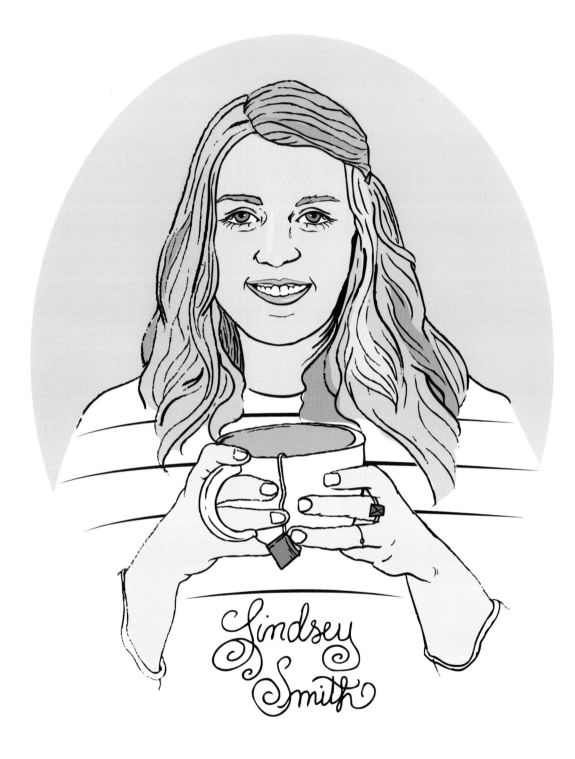

Lindsey Smith

INTRODUCTION

Hiya!

What started as just another Tuesday morning in September, with my normal morning meditation routine, turned into stress city by midafternoon. Between coaching students, answering emails, and dealing with the daily tasks of being a human, I had had enough adulting for one day. However, since it was only noon and I still had a million things on my to-do list, I had no choice but to trudge forward.

At about two p.m., I was mentally spent, stressed, and feeling blue. The second I sat back in my chair to take a break, I felt an urge come upon me.

I needed chocolate—and I needed it immediately.

I ventured downstairs to see what kind of confections I could find in my pantry. As soon as I passed my dining room, before I even made it to the kitchen, I saw my husband look up at me with what I only remember as a questioning look. It was as if he knew what I was about to do.

Instead of hiding it, I looked over and said, "Yes, I'm eating my feelings right now," and proceeded to walk into the kitchen to grab a dose of dark chocolate.

As I made my way out of the kitchen, I caught another glimpse of him before I hit the stairs to go back to my office and casually mumbled, "Don't judge me."

The words "don't judge me" used to echo in my subconscious after I ate something I didn't think I should be eating. I carried guilt into every food I felt like I shouldn't have and typically felt worse after eating anything I labeled as "bad." Sure, I felt good temporarily. After a candy bar, I felt like I could conquer the world. An hour later, though, I felt dead to the world. This roller-coaster relationship with food could only last so long before something needed to change.

The way I eat my feelings now is much different from how I ate my feelings when I was growing up. I used to use "bad food" as a reward system. If I went to the gym, I deserved a pizza, and when I started to write, if I wrote two thousand words, I would get some chocolate. I sometimes would pretend I was competing at the Olympics, except the game was normal life tasks and the prize was Sour Patch gummies, the holy grail of food rewards.

It wasn't until I stopped and actually listened to what my body was telling me that I realized that what we eat greatly impacts how we feel—and also how we feel can impact what we eat. Most times a piece of kale will not be able to fix a heartbreak, just like chocolate is not the answer to all your problems at work. (Sorry if you are just finding this out!) Sometimes we need nourishment beyond food and should incorporate what I call "lifestyle foods" in our diet. So maybe kale won't fix your heartache, but a listening ear might help start the healing process. I learned that if you allow yourself to dig just a little bit deeper and learn to feel your feelings rather than stuff

them, you can actually find out what you are lacking that food can't possibly solve.

Once you get to know your body, you will begin to understand that you can truly "eat your feelings" for the benefit of your body and mind—and not just as a temporary mood stabilizer that usually results in a worse mood later on.

Instead of looking at food as "good" or "bad," you will instead learn to simply nourish your body with foods that make you feel good. Sometimes it's healthy greens and proteins and other times you might just want that chocolate brownie.

So when I say "eat your feelings," what I mean is that if you are feeling sad, stressed, exhausted, hangry, or bored, you can find comfort in dishes you love and tend to gravitate toward or crave. But instead of processed ingredients, you can make them with mood-boosting ingredients that will nourish you physically.

It's okay to feel sad and gravitate toward something like ice cream. This book gives you the opportunity to do that—and simultaneously improve your mood.

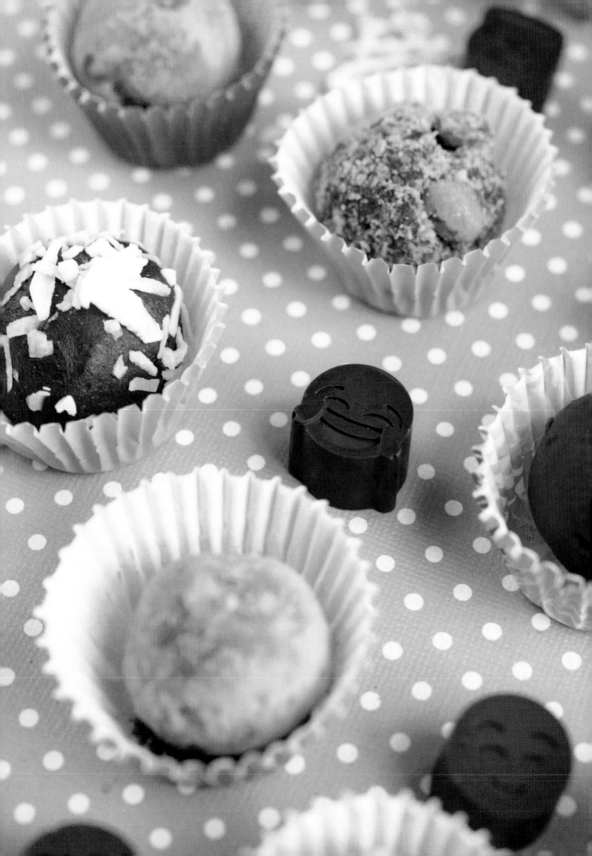

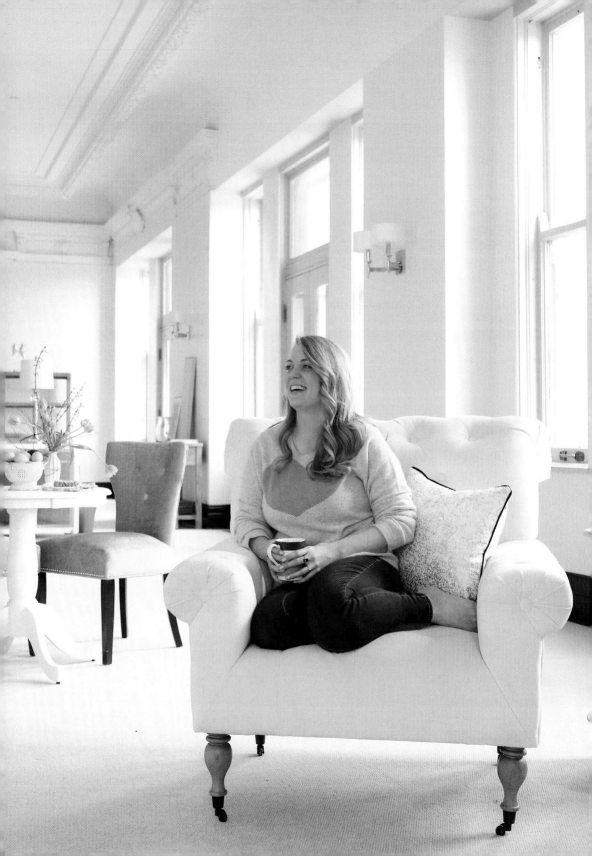

one

THE FOOD MOOD FEMIFESTO

I f you are reading this, you are a miracle. That puts you right up there with the Pyramids of Giza, Machu Picchu, the Taj Mahal, and cheese. (Seriously, have you had a creamy hunk of smoked Gouda before? That is what I call miraculous.)

Your body is like a magical machine that is constantly working for you and through you. It breathes without reminders to do so. Its heart beats to keep you alive. Yes, it even digests that half-chewed candy bar you scarfed down while you were hangry. And it did it all with love, hoping for nothing but the best results in keeping you happy, healthy, and alive.

When it comes to food and your body, the Food Mood Lifestyle is one that honors your unique body. Every shape, size, and style is to be celebrated, not shamed. It's one where your mental health has more value than a carefully orchestrated Instagram photo ever will. It's about eating good and healthy food because you love your body, not because you don't.

The Food Mood Lifestyle believes that your food choices impact your mood as much as your mood impacts your food choices. More important, the Food Mood Lifestyle recognizes that food provides physical nutrients as well as emotional and spiritual nutrients. Some days, a kale juice gives your body the nutrients it needs. Other days, no food can substitute for a friend, loved one, or coworker giving you a hug or telling you that you are valued. And sometimes, you just want a damn piece of chocolate cake, without guilt and with all the love.

There is always room for pure comfort. Sometimes no matter how hard you try to re-create Grandma's apple pie, it's not actually Grandma's Apple Pie. So in those moments, indulge in the real thing, without guilt and with all the love. And now when I go for that dark chocolate, it's because I'm listening to my body and truly eating my feelings for the benefit of my body, not for an emotional escape. I instead eat chocolate because it contains ingredients that can help physically nourish my mind and improve my mood. Your body will thank you when you give it what it needs.

The Food Mood Lifestyle does not judge. It believes that everyone is on their own unique journey and path. We need our stories, experiences, ups, and downs to take us along the path, to feel the feelings of life, and to savor the magic that is within us.

The Food Mood Lifestyle trusts. It trusts the wisdom of your unique body, realizing that if you listen carefully, the answers will be given to you. Your gut instinct is almost always right. Trust yourself every day.

And lastly, the Food Mood Lifestyle loves. It believes that self-love is the most nutrient-dense vitamin available. By loving yourself and fueling up on self-love, you can rid yourself of hanger pangs and learn to love others fully. Treat your body with respect. Talk to your body as you would talk to someone you love and appreciate. Love it greatly. Cherish it fully. Your body is the only one you have, so love it up the best you can while you can.

Check out the full femifesto on pages 8 and 9.

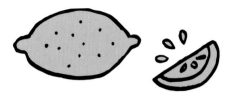

Create Your Food Mood Morning Routine

Having a solid morning routine can help you accomplish more, feel more productive, and incorporate your personal health and happiness into your everyday life.

Here are some ways in which you can have a solid healthy morning routine:

- **Plan the night before.** Review your calendar, create a task list, and have an idea of what you are doing the next day. This will help set your morning up for success.

- **Give yourself time.** Allow at least fifteen minutes in the morning dedicated to you. Maybe do some writing, meditate, or just simply have some peace and quiet to yourself. Build this into your routine.

- **Set an intention.** While you are lying in bed, right before you are about to get up, set an intention for the day. Maybe say to yourself, "I want to be filled with joy today" or "I want to bring others joy." Or maybe your intention is focused around an area of your life such as "I want to create amazing opportunities for my business today" or "I want to be healthy today." Whatever your intention is, start your day with one that speaks to you and allow it to carry through the day.

- **Make your bed.** Creating an orderly space before you leave for the day can help you reduce your stress levels later on. When you come home to sleep at night, slipping into a neatly made bed will make you feel relaxed and calm.

- **Drink warm lemon water.** Warm lemon water can help give your body an energizing burst, wake you up faster, and get your digestive tract in tune for the day.

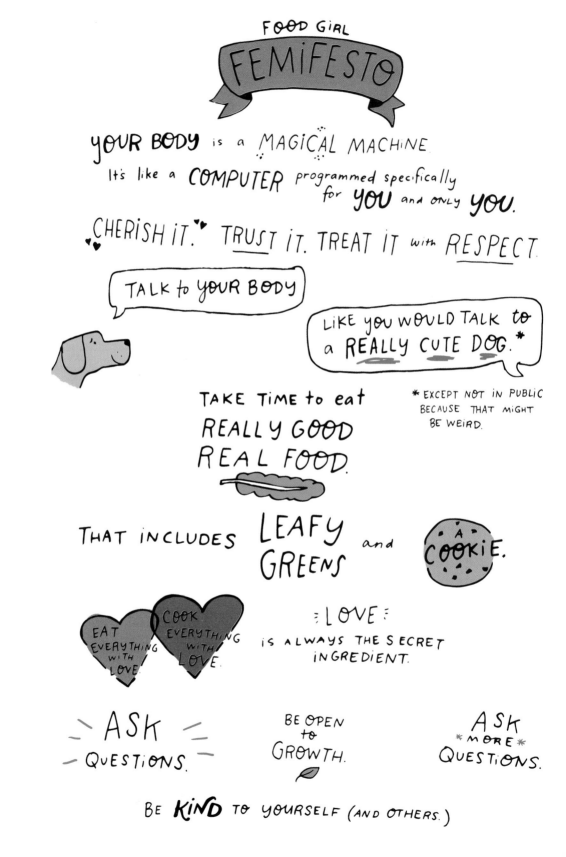

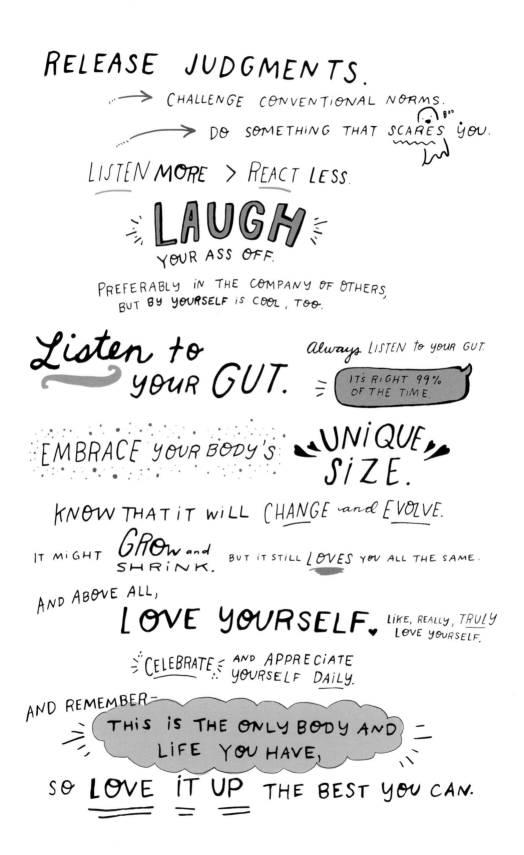

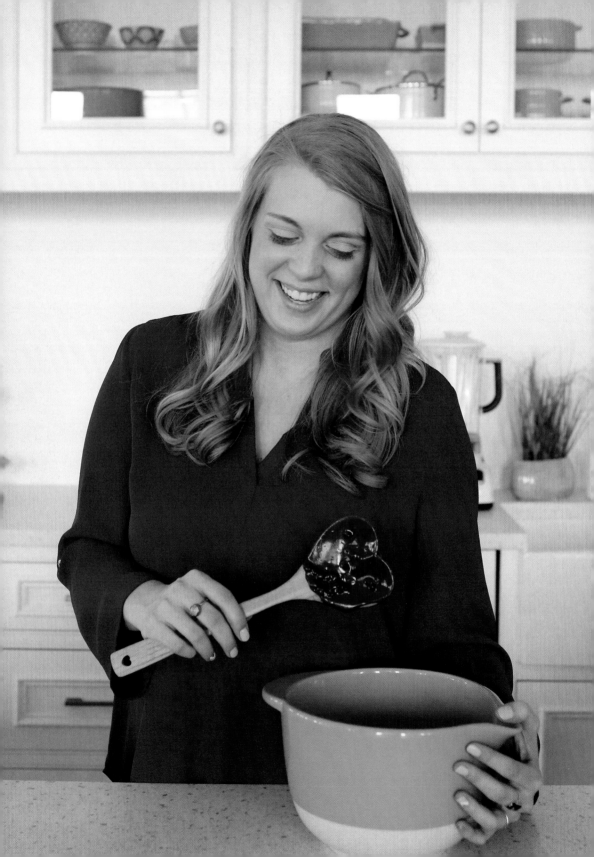

two

UNDERSTANDING YOUR FOOD MOOD

The Roller-Coaster Emotions of Food

In college, I lived for the weekends when I had no more classes and more freedom to do what I wanted.

I loved having girls' nights, getting dressed up and going out for a night on the town. All week I anticipated the freedom that no work or classes would bring.

By the time Friday came, I had my outfit prepped, shoes ready, and eyebrow game on point. (Just kidding, they probably looked a mess, but that makes me sound cooler.)

However, there was one big thing missing from my day: food.

I was so obsessed with looking good and "feeling skinny" on a night out on the town that I would purposefully starve myself all day so I could go out and feel thin. I would maybe eat a really small breakfast—like a granola bar and some water—but for the rest of the day, food was off limits.

By seven p.m., I was so hangry that it was hard to have a good time.

This type of disordered eating is no way to live. Not only was I depriving my body of the nutrients and minerals it needed to sustain itself, but I actually thought not eating would make me happier about my appearance—which it never did.

Our relationship with food is often so complex. We all have relationships with food that stem from our parents, great-grandparents, peers, teachers, the media, our school cafeteria, and food advertisements.

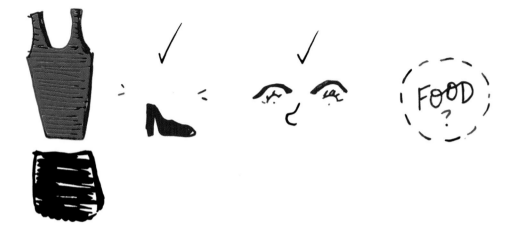

Many times, we think we are doing right by our body, but often we are just causing our body and our mental health more harm than good.

Here are just some of the reasons we eat (or don't eat):

Unrealistic Dieting: Are you on the all-carb, no-carb, or some-carb diet? Maybe you eat nothing but meat for days on end? Or nothing but vegetables until you start looking like a carrot? Whether you try paleo, vegetarian, Atkins, the sushi diet, the raw food diet, or the "you name it, let's sell it" diet, many times these diets can wreak havoc on your body . . . because let's face it: every BODY is different. You read that right. What works for Susie in accounting might not work the same for you. And while it's great to think that cutting those calories and replacing them with five 100-calorie packs a day will do the trick, you may be, in fact, perpetuating the emotional turmoil that unrealistic dieting can cause. Avoid diets like the Green Tea Pill diet, the Nothing But Water diet, the Lean Cuisine diet, or anything that is sold on an infomercial or at Big Lots.

Deprivation: Have you ever gone to a party and feared the dessert table? After all, desserts are pretty much the devil and go straight to your thighs, butt, stomach, hips—you name it. And while you are hanging out by the water and carrot sticks, it seems as if all your friends are eating what they want, drinking, and being merry. You feel like old Scrooge. That's because deprivation (yes, even of those sweet or salty treats) can trigger food binges later on. When you deprive yourself throughout the day, you naturally want to overcompensate later. Physically, your body is depleted of essential nutrients when you deprive yourself, which then leads to emotional chaos. Your body is attempting to seek justice because it doesn't feel it was properly served at the party, hence the food binges later. Constantly returning to deprivation is like the definition of insanity often attributed to Einstein: doing the same thing over and over again and expecting a different result. Deprivation never made anyone happy, just hangry.

Indecisive Food Choices: Do you ever have those days when you don't really crave anything in particular? You start asking yourself questions like "Wait, do I want a salad or soup? A chicken salad or a beet salad? Or should I just get a veggie sandwich?" Maybe you decide not to eat anything. Being indecisive about food choices can actually increase your chances of not eating anything at all. And not eating anything at all is the most surefire way to end up bingeing later on.

Undereating: Coffee for breakfast? Check! Small salad for lunch? Check! An apple for a snack? Check! Some broccoli and a small piece of lean chicken for dinner? Check! Nine p.m.: Hangry? Double check! Even when we think we are eating enough throughout the day, chances are we are not. Even though the "calories in, calories out" myth has been debunked, we are still a calorie-obsessed culture. Just because you are eating food (even healthy food) doesn't necessarily mean you are eating enough of it. And when you don't eat enough, your body starts slowly going into starvation mode, so by the time nine p.m. comes around, you become a raging, hangry beast who just wants a snack! Instead, you eat one container of hummus, two slices of pizza, and some fro-yo. Whoops.

Overworking/Skipped Meals: Do you ever get wrapped up in a project only to find yourself way past the lunch hour? You think to yourself, "I'm not that hungry, I can wait a couple more hours until dinner." Or maybe you intentionally skip a meal because you want to look good in your dress for tonight's date. Then another hour or so goes by and you find yourself full of rage, trying to hold back the tears? That's because skipping meals can cause major ugly-crying episodes later. Even if you don't feel that hungry, hunger can creep up on you and creep up fast in between meals, especially if you skip them. You can only trick your mind into being busy for so long before the hunger pangs and coffee shakes start to creep in.

Stress: Nearly 77 percent of Americans regularly experience physical symptoms caused by stress. Stress can affect everything from sleep and energy to digestion and brain function. It's safe to say that stress is a major underlying cause for many diseases. When you are feeling stressed or emotionally and physically drained, normally the last thing you want to do is prepare something to eat or go grocery shopping. So instead you opt for Netflix and forget that food doesn't make itself. This decision takes your stressed-out, grumpy attitude and puts it on blast as your fooditude starts to unleash.

Lack of Preparation: Do you usually have good intentions to start off the week? Like "Okay, on Sunday, I am going to prepare all my meals for the week." Sunday rolls around and you find yourself too lazy or hungover (or both), and suddenly those lofty preparation goals fall by the wayside as "Netflix and chill" seems like a way better use of your time. (Oh, wait, we mean the actual "Netflix and chill," as in you binge-watch copious amounts of *Unbreakable Kimmy Schmidt* in sweatpants on the couch.) Hanger can happen when we just simply aren't prepared. We forget that food is a priority and not an option.

We Were Born This Way (Why We Emotionally Eat)

Let's think about the evolution of food and eating.

Our cavemen and -women ancestors did whatever it took to get their next meal because, quite frankly, they didn't know if or when it would come. They hunted wild animals and gathered what they could scavenge. They were truly hunting and eating to survive. This made food something extremely emotional. I don't know about you, but chasing a wild animal in hopes it doesn't kill me first would tend to keep me a bit . . . stressed. By "stressed" I really mean I would be a crumbling emotional mess.

Now think about newborn babies. If they are hungry, they cry. Need a drink? They cry. Want a snack? They whine and throw a hanger tantrum. From day one, children use their emotions to let those around them know when they are hungry or thirsty.

As babies evolve into toddlers and grade-schoolers, food not only sustains them and keeps them full, but they also start experimenting with the emotions foods bring them. It's not uncommon for children to cry for a certain snack when they get older or to become almost dependent on certain foods that give them comfort. Suddenly, chicken soup becomes a sick day staple and Grandma's cookies are a must-have upon entering her house.

And then we become adults. And damn it, adulting is hard. And suddenly, the world seems to move faster, we tend to gravitate toward convenient foods, and we emotionally eat everything except the foods that will actually help us with said emotion. Happy? Want to celebrate? Eat! Sad? Need to be consoled? Food! Hangry? Anything will do! Tired? Grab a coffee. Bored? Pizza looks good.

For every emotion, we can pick a food that we think deserves our full attention.

And this impulse makes sense. Food gives us a sense of pleasure and joy. It can provide us with satisfaction and comfort. Food can awaken each of our senses to something new each time we eat. It gives us energy and quite literally sustains life as we know it. It should be emotional.

However, in modern times, emotional eating is no longer a necessity. Sure, we still need food to survive, but we don't carry the same animalistic instincts we did as cave people. Instead, emotional eating has become a luxury and not a mere necessity.

Instead of looking at food as a sustaining and pleasurable experience,

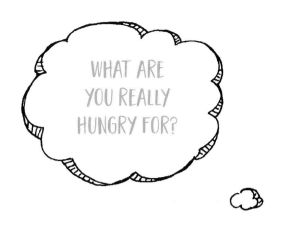

WHAT ARE YOU REALLY HUNGRY FOR?

we now use our innate emotional eating skills to escape from stress, sadness, or any sort of negative feeling. Often it's not the food that we really want. We're chasing a deep emotional desire that food alone cannot possibly fix.

It's okay to be an emotional eater. After all, we were born that way. Instead of beating yourself up over the fact that you are attempting to find bliss in a bag of Doritos, instead start to ask yourself this one big question:

What are you really hungry for?

When you stop and ask yourself this question, you realize we tend to turn to food in times of emotional crisis—yet the one thing we really need isn't food at all.

And sure, sometimes the answer to "What are you hungry for?" *is* that ice cream sundae or some chips. But if you allow yourself to dig a little deeper, you will often find that it is emotional sustenance you have really been craving

COMMON CRAVINGS	WHAT YOUR BODY MAY REALLY NEED	SAMPLE NUTRIENTS TO INCORPORATE	EAT YOUR FEELINGS RECIPES
SWEET FOOD	Natural energy Less red meat Detoxifying nutrients Less stress More rest Balance	Dark leafy greens Fish such as salmon and trout Berries such as blueberries, strawberries, or raspberries Sweet vegetables like carrots and sweet potatoes Natural sweeteners like maple syrup or stevia More sleep/rest Quiet meditation Time with friends and family	Cookie Dough Contraband (159) Sweet Potato Chips (179) Easy Creamy Spinach (199) Date Night Bites (219) Green Boredom Smoothie (254)
SALTY FOOD	Natural minerals More water	Natural, unrefined sea salt Root vegetables like carrots, beets, and potatoes High water content foods like cucumber, pineapples, celery, strawberries, and watermelon Sea vegetables	Easy Hand Roll (147) Sage Sweet Potato and Asparagus Risotto (137) Berry Burst Smoothie (209) Cucumber Cups (229) Zucchini Pasta (246)
CHOCOLATE	Magnesium Stable blood sugar Balance	Raw nuts, seeds, and legumes Fruits such as cherries, grapefruits, apples, and pears Natural sweeteners like agave nectar or stevia Exercise Stress-reducing activities like reading, writing, and yoga	Dark Chocolate + Sea Salt Brownies (131) Raspberry Bites (160) Go-To Quinoa Salad (206) Cinnamon Pear Salad (225) Chocolate Almond Tartlets (237)
CAFFEINE	Natural energy Less stress More rest Balance Detoxifying nutrients Exercise	Dark leafy greens Raw fruits Raw nuts, seeds, and legumes Brown rice, quinoa, barley, and other whole grains	Avocado Toast (146) Iced Turmeric Lemonade (183) Easy Energy Bars (191) Power Wrap (230) Crispy Chickpeas (251)
BREAD/PASTA	Whole grains Balance	Brown rice pasta Cauliflower or potatoes Raw nuts, seeds, and legumes Brown rice, quinoa, and barley Time with friends and family A daily gratitude practice	Mushroom Melt Skillet (143) Spaghetti Squash Bake (179) Mini Quiches (195) Almond Chia Bread (229) Rosemary Cheese Crackers (253)

Own Your Food Cravings

We look at cravings, especially those pesky emotional eating cravings, as a "bad" thing.

"Oh no, I cannot believe I am craving ice cream. WHY! I haven't craved ice cream in years because I've been eating so well. Now all of a sudden I want not just ice cream but a sundae with whipped cream, sprinkles, and hot fudge."

You then convince yourself that you shouldn't have the sundae because you will gain fifty pounds after eating just one. So you settle for some ice cubes in your water instead.

"I mean, it's cold, just like ice cream. And if I pretend hard enough, I can taste the sprinkles."

No. Just no.

Rather than disowning your cravings, you need to OWN them instead. Listen to them. Anytime you get a craving, say, "YES! Now I have a chance to learn more about myself and my body," instead of immediately dismissing it. When you dismiss your cravings, you miss an opportunity to explore what your body needs.

I remember one time I was really craving a chocolate brownie. I told myself, "No, Lindsey, you cannot have a chocolate brownie. That's bad."

So I had a couple of pieces of dark chocolate instead. An hour later, I was still thinking about that brownie. But I kept telling myself I couldn't have it. Well, a bar of dark chocolate, two gluten-free cookies, some cheese bread, and a failed "healthy" hot chocolate later . . . I still just wanted that damn brownie.

I then thought to myself, "What if I just allowed myself to eat the one brownie I really wanted?" I not only would have avoided eating a mix of the most random and unfulfilling things, but I would have eaten the brownie, enjoyed it, and then moved on with my day.

When you dismiss your cravings, not only are you robbing yourself of the opportunity to learn and grow, but those feelings are then replaced with guilt, sadness, and dissatisfaction. Cravings are the gatekeepers that unlock the secrets to our unique bodies.

So the next time you crave something, try digging deeper to see why you are craving it.

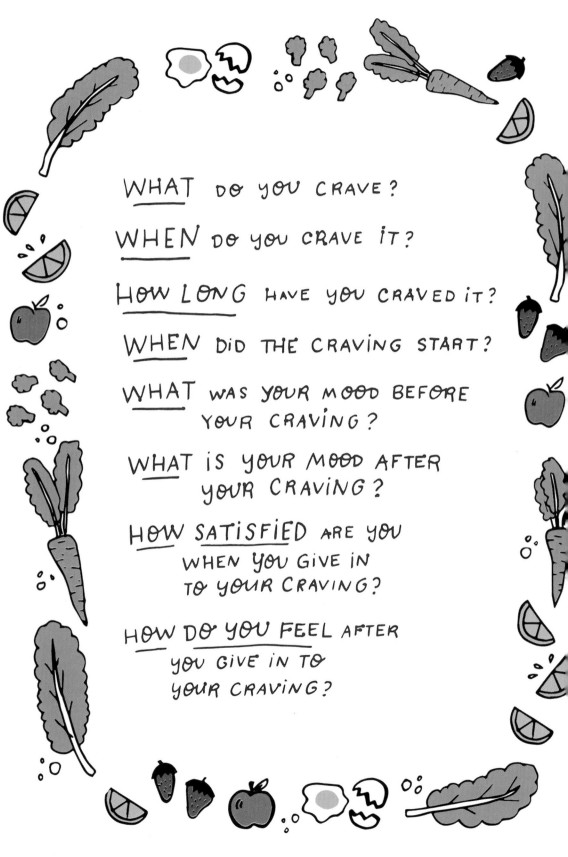

WHAT DO YOU CRAVE?

WHEN DO YOU CRAVE IT?

HOW LONG HAVE YOU CRAVED IT?

WHEN DID THE CRAVING START?

WHAT WAS YOUR MOOD BEFORE
YOUR CRAVING?

WHAT IS YOUR MOOD AFTER
YOUR CRAVING?

HOW SATISFIED ARE YOU
WHEN YOU GIVE IN
TO YOUR CRAVING?

HOW DO YOU FEEL AFTER
YOU GIVE IN TO
YOUR CRAVING?

What Your Cravings REALLY Mean

Once you are open to understanding your cravings, it's important to dig deeper to process what they are really trying to tell you. I don't mean whispering into a jar of peanut butter, "Peanut butter, my friend, why am I craving you right now?" I mean, you CAN ask that question, but try to do it discreetly and with less drama.

Every craving can tell you something specific about your physical or emotional needs—you just need to start listening.

For example, craving sweet food could mean that you are eating a diet high in red meat and maybe you should lay off the steaks for a bit in order to restore balance and curb your sugar cravings. It could also mean that you are craving some sweetness from life itself and need a fun night out with friends or a night in by yourself to bake a batch of cookies. If you are craving salty food, your body might be lacking some essential minerals found in sea salt. It could also mean you're really craving memories of those carnivals and festivals where you enjoyed fries as a kid.

Understanding your cravings is both a science and an art form. From a science standpoint, there are reasons your body craves certain foods when it does. Many times it can be a mineral deficiency or an overconsumption of a certain food.

And from an art standpoint, cravings are much like an intricate dance that you and only you can choreograph. It's usually not so much about the physical food you need but more about the "life nutrients" your body is craving.

The chart on page 16 shows the most common cravings we have, complete with what your body may really need. And remember, sometimes your body needs beef jerky as much as it needs balance. Keep listening and you will soon discover your unique craving patterns.

> **Reduce Your Cravings Every Time You Brush!**
>
> Tongue cleaners are an underrated tool that can help not just keep your breath smelling fresh but also remove bacteria and food particles, which can help reduce food cravings and awaken your taste buds to new foods and flavors.

The Deeper Side of Cravings

Physical food cravings are actually so intricately wrapped up in our DNA and emotional intelligence that, often, a simple vegetable or fruit can't kick it. We have cravings for more than just physical reasons.

OUR ANCESTRY

Although we don't entirely understand them, our genes and physical makeup have been passed down from generation to generation. This includes not only health issues and looks but also emotional traits. Whether you know it or not, your random craving for sauerkraut can be embedded deep within your ancestral lineage.

Getting to know and understand your heritage and what came before you can help give you a glimpse into your own health, quirks, and personality.

I had this experience when I was randomly flipping through my cable TV channels and I caught an episode about ancestry. The researchers traced people's ancestry and showed them their family backgrounds, including where they came from, what their ancestors' jobs were, what their heritage was, and sometimes even a glimpse into their familys' personalities. I was never too much into my own ancestry until I saw this episode. After I saw it, I immediately signed up for every website related to ancestry and was even two seconds away from booking a flight to the ancestry library in Utah. I spent five hours pulling my ancestry together and eventually had to stop when I found that one of my great-grandparents was named John Smith and I couldn't go down the rabbit hole any further. I did learn that I am a fourth-generation business owner in my family. My great-great-grandpap emigrated here from Germany and started a small convenience store. His son followed suit. And then my grandma and grandpa started their own corner store, and eventually my parents opened a flooring store. And here I am, an entrepreneurial spirit in my nature and, I like to think, my DNA. There was something that carried through into my genes to give me the sense that I have.

Once I uncovered my entrepreneurial DNA, I decided to dig a little bit deeper into my ancestry to understand my health and cravings. I took a closer look at where I came from and how the foods I gravitate toward and crave could have to do with my ancestry. Not only did I realize I have one of the highest DNA markers that could be traced back to Neanderthals (cavewoman status!), but I also got to see where in the world my family immigrated to America from. Aside from learning about my cavewoman heritage, my DNA also showcased that most of my ancestors came from Britain and Ireland.

Suddenly, thanks to my British heritage, my love of tea (I've been drinking it since I was a kid!) made perfect sense. However, the most fascinating thing of all was to find out that I was likely to have a high tolerance for dairy. People who are of Irish descent tend to have a genetic trait that makes them able to easily digest dairy. Since Ireland is known for its dairy farms, which have been a staple of their culture, Irish bodies have adapted to dairy, producing specific enzymes to help break it down. It was amazing to think that my own health can be traced back to generations and generations of people with different ethnicities. It's incredible and shows how amazing the body truly is.

Since everyone has a unique DNA makeup, it's no wonder we are all so different and respond to different foods in different ways. Understanding your own unique DNA can give you a glimpse into not just where you come from, but also personality quirks and health traits.

THE SEASONS

Your neighborhood, the climate, and the change (or lack of change) of the seasons can all greatly impact your cravings. For example, if you live in a climate with four seasons and changing weather, your body might crave different foods at different times of the year. You might join the bandwagon with everyone and crave pumpkin spice everything as soon as fall hits. Or on the first hot day of summer, you might find yourself jonesin' for some ice cream. This is because as the seasons change, our nutritional needs change. We want warming foods in the fall and winter, while the spring and summer tend to demand lighter and colder foods. If you live in the Bahamas, the foods you crave are probably going to be a lot different than if you live in Iceland.

EMOTIONAL MEMORIES

Feelings associated with holidays, seasons, or even certain days of the week can also trigger memories that can lead us down a craving path. For example, if you lost a loved one around a certain season or on a certain type of day (like rainy or foggy), those emotions might flare up when it rains or becomes foggy. You might notice that you seem to feel sad for no real reason, but in reality you have a deep emotional memory. Oftentimes, we can turn to food or even a certain type of food to make us feel better.

There are also emotional elements when it comes to the changing seasons, depending on what you experienced during that time. And if you find yourself craving ice cream in the winter, you might really be craving something emotional that the feeling of summer or another specific time gives you.

When I lost my dad to cancer, it was a rainy day on the weekend. For the next year, during rainy weekends, I always craved a grilled cheese. I realized that the reason I craved a grilled cheese was because on rainy weekends when I was growing up, my dad and I would eat grilled cheese and watch *Unsolved Mysteries*. I quickly realized that it wasn't the grilled cheese I was truly craving; it was time with my dad that I wanted.

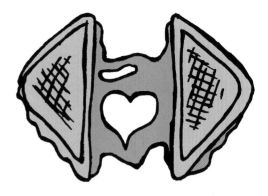

A grilled cheese wasn't going to bring my dad back, so instead, I found other ways to honor my dad's memory when I got that memory craving. Sometimes I would go do a random act of kindness for someone since my dad was always doing that, and other times I would put on an episode of *Unsolved Mysteries*. When you can nourish your cravings in ways food can't, many times you will feel much more satisfied.

HORMONES

Hormones directly impact our food cravings. A week before women get their period, they might find themselves craving iron-rich foods like beef or proteins. You might also crave chocolate because your body is lacking magnesium. Understanding how your specific hormones work can help alleviate cravings, or you can know what you need to feed it properly.

I went vegan for about a year, and I

noticed that a week before my period I would get sick. At one point, I felt weak and passed out. I also happened to be craving red meat, which I hadn't eaten in almost five years. I resisted this craving because I thought I could be stronger than it, but I only got sicker as the months moved on. Eventually, I decided to listen to my body and ate a grass-fed burger a week before my period. Not only did it taste delicious, but those low-iron symptoms vanished. Now that I know my body and my cycle, I make sure to include iron-rich foods such as lentils, nuts, seeds, greens, and quinoa to better prepare for those low-iron weeks.

SELF-SABOTAGING SYNDROME

As humans, we are constantly seeking balance. We want things to be smooth and even. However, if things are going really well, our initial instinct is to think that this is too good to be true. This can lead to self-sabotage. Have you ever eaten healthy all week, only to realize all the fun got sucked out of food choices, leading you to binge-eat cookies and snacks on Friday at nine p.m. just to try to restore some sort of balance to the universe? That's self-sabotaging syndrome at its finest. When things are going really well, we often freak out. We do this in relationships (have you ever broken up with someone because it was too good to seem real?!)—and we do this with food.

When this type of emotion takes control, stop to see if you notice a pattern. For example, every time you say you are going to diet, do you end up sneaking food into your room late at night so no one sees? If you do this every time you declare a diet, maybe you shouldn't declare a diet anymore, but instead say, "I want to get healthy." Shifting something this simple can help your self-sabotaging syndrome disappear.

Be Your Own Food-Mood-Etarian

In 2011, I was giving one of my first-ever lectures on emotional eating, and after the talk I asked the audience if anyone had any questions. One young woman raised her hand and asked, "I know you said we need to listen to our own bodies, but I want to know, what type of diet do you eat?"

People ask me this question most often—and I understand why. If we see something work for someone else, we want to try it. That's why there are all kinds of weird crazes and obsessions each year with kids' toys. It can be the dumbest toy ever, but suddenly, it's the hot item and everyone wants it.

I feel this same way about diets. Why have 99 percent of people tried a diet at one point in their lives? They see what other people "have"—whether it's flat abs, weight loss, or less anxiety—and they want that, too.

When someone first asked me this, I nervously responded that I was a vegetarian with some exceptions, and then proceeded to list things I didn't eat. Then I explained that sometimes I eat fish. And I love dark chocolate.

The reason for my long-winded and half-assed answer partly had to do with nerves of a newbie speaker, but also because I didn't want this young woman to think that my way of eating was necessarily the best for her, her mood, and her body. I also knew that the statistics would not work in my favor. While 99 percent of people attempt a diet, only 2 percent actually succeed with their weight-loss and diet goals. As a nutrition coach, I feel I have a moral obligation to assist people in finding what works for them, not give them the prescription for *my* unique body's needs.

After I left that conference, I kept wondering how I could address this question whenever it came up. When the Q&A at the next conference came along, like clockwork, someone again asked me the same familiar question.

Immediately my mind went blank and I could feel my throat closing up. I wondered if I should bare all and give them a copy of my food journal or if I should ask them why they even care.

This time, I laughed and responded, "I'm a food-mood-etarian. I eat what makes me feel good and makes me happy."

So there you have it. A food-mood-etarian was born. Whether you are plant-based or paleo, Atkins or raw food, food-mood-etarianism is one lifestyle that works for everyone.

Being a food-mood-etarian is not a fancy diet or strict plan that you follow for a month and then never look at again. It's not a fad, and honestly, it's not even that glamorous. It will evolve and change as your body does, and you'll have to do the detective work to figure it out. But guess what? It's your plan and your blueprint for your unique body. It helps you dig deep and discover who you really are. It helps you find out what you crave and what your body needs. It helps you feel your feelings, eat your feelings, and have a good time doing it.

Being a food-mood-etarian is a way of life.

No Scale Needed

I will be honest: it only takes one look at the scale for me to turn into an anxiety-ridden mess with low self-esteem for weeks.

With a five-foot, four-inch frame, weighing in at 145 pounds, I often used to feel defeated about my weight. I would constantly obsess over getting back to my high school weight of 130 pounds, and anytime I saw the scale stray from that weight, I was left feeling not good enough.

While today I feel happy, healthy, and truly good in my body, I spent so many years obsessed over that number. For what?

In America we like to measure things. We like transactions. We like to know that if we do X, then we will get Y as a result. And we certainly love to define both things and people by size, appearance, and financial success.

Weight is just another measurement in our culture. If we are overweight, we are less-than. If we are underweight, we are less-than. We have to have the "perfect" look and weight in order to feel a sense of worth. And sometimes even then we fall short.

But should weight be the overarching determining factor in whether you are healthy? Should we still be defining our self-worth by a number on the scale? Or, even more, should we still be defining our *health* as a number on a scale?

When it comes down to it, weight should be a factor of how we view health. Sure, certain numbers can tell us a whole heck of a lot about our health. But numbers can't tell us how we feel emotionally, physically, or spiritually. Numbers cannot tell us how our bodies feel.

So, instead of weighing yourself, I challenge you to measure your health in these other ways:

ENERGY LEVEL

Do you have plenty of energy, or are you constantly feeling fatigued? Your energy level is a huge indicator of your overall health and well-being. Strive to feel energetic in your body by fueling yourself rather than depriving yourself.

HOW YOU REALLY FEEL IN YOUR BODY

This is a big one. Make sure to ask yourself how you really feel. It's important to dig deep to understand your body's unique cravings and needs. Many times, we can be the weight we always dreamed of but still be sick and unhealthy. Always check in with your health by simply analyzing how you feel in your body.

DIGESTION

Your health starts in your gut, so it's important to make sure it's functioning properly. Is your digestion on track? (This is the technical way of asking, "Are you pooping regularly?") A key indicator to good health is a healthy digestive tract. So make sure it's properly functioning by fueling your gut with probiotics (kombucha, anyone?), whole grains, and whole foods.

YOUR JEANS

Women especially lose inches before pounds, so rather than rely on a scale, rely on your jeans for a more accurate reading. How do they fit? Do they feel looser? Or just right? Notice how your jeans fit when you feel your best and aim for that!

SELF-LOVE

Last but not least, how well are you treating or loving yourself? Are you constantly beating yourself up or tearing yourself apart? Negative self-inflicted behaviors can be just as toxic as processed food. It's important to clear your head space and practice self-love because not only does your health depend on it, your body deserves it.

The Technical Side of Food and Mood

It's time to get technical. And by "technical" I mean as sciency as someone who likes to swear and prefers explanations for stuff in the form of dog videos over textbook definitions can get.

Now that you know about food-mood-etarianism, it's time to start uncovering the food-mood connection. In this section, you'll learn about the brain-gut connection, important neurotransmitters, foods that deflate your mood, and a complete list of mood-boosting foods and what they are good for.

As you move through this section, remember that your body is uniquely made. Only you can determine which foods make you feel good and which ones don't. Everybody is different—so take that into account as you learn more about your own food moods.

LISTEN TO YOUR GUT

Have you ever experienced those nervous and anxious butterflies in your stomach when you know something is oh-so-wrong? Or maybe you have experienced that "gut reaction" or "gut

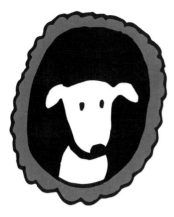

instinct" to something you know is oh-so-right? Well, there is an actual reason for that that isn't just folklore. Your gut, often referred to as your "second brain," is actually your first responder to stress. This is the reason it gives you those funky feelings when something doesn't seem right or those butterflies when you go on a first date with someone extra cute. Or, in my case, anytime I see an adorable photo of my dog.

Your digestive tract contains more than 100 million nerve cells. These cells, known as the enteric nervous system, communicate directly with your brain. Unlike your actual brain, your gut can't debate politics with your in-laws, but it does feel the initial stress response from those debates and sends signals to your nervous system, hormones, and immune system to let them know that Aunt Sally's new political bumper stickers are not going over so well. This constant stress response in the gut eventually increases cortisol levels, weakens the immune

system, and sometimes leads to chronic inflammation or pain.

Any type of stress, whether it's good or bad, can cause your body to move into a state of fight or flight. If you are watching a scary movie and something unexpected causes you to jump, your body will feel the stress and the knots in your stomach. Eventually, however, you will realize it was a fake scary movie and your body will return to normal.

When you experience low levels of stress on a daily basis, combined with the occasionally anxiety-inducing scary movies, your body has to work harder to normalize. If the stress is chronic, it can lead to chronic inflammation. At first, you might experience physical symptoms in your gut such as indigestion, acid reflux, constipation, weight gain, or an upset stomach. But eventually chronic inflammation can also affect your mood, causing anxiety, depression, and other mood disorders.

So when it comes to your gut, it's important to treat it with respect by honoring your gut instinct, both physically and mentally. If something feels off, listen to your gut. If something feels right, go with your gut. And if something makes your gut physically ill, listen and adjust your diet.

Your body is an incredible machine, remember? The best thing you can do for your health is listen to it.

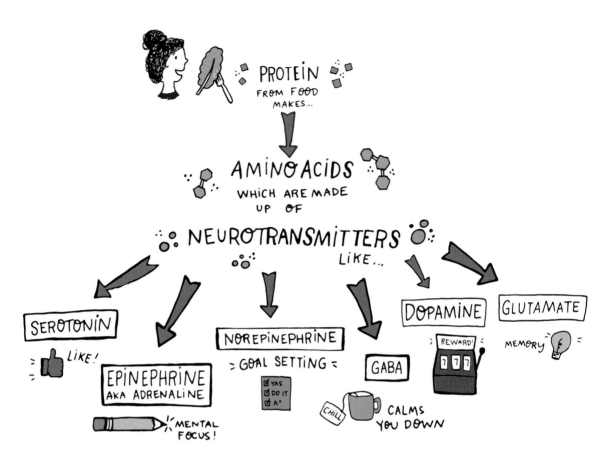

PROTEIN
FROM FOOD
MAKES...

AMINO ACIDS
WHICH ARE MADE
UP OF

NEUROTRANSMITTERS
LIKE...

SEROTONIN
LIKE!

EPINEPHRINE
AKA ADRENALINE
MENTAL FOCUS!

NOREPINEPHRINE
GOAL SETTING
☑ YAS
☑ DO IT
☑ A*

GABA
CHILL
CALMS YOU DOWN

DOPAMINE
REWARD!
7 7 7

GLUTAMATE
MEMORY

THE NEUROTRANSMITTERS YOU NEED TO KNOW

Neurotransmitters are brain chemicals that release and send communications through the body and brain. Certain neurotransmitters are crucial for balancing moods, and if they aren't functioning properly, they can cause mood disorders such as anxiety and depression.

Here is a simple breakdown of how neurotransmitters work:

When protein is processed, it makes amino acids. (Imagine crunching on some spinach salad.) Amino acids are made up of neurotransmitters. These neurotransmitters act as chemical hormones and can help regulate mood and sleep. Your body needs a balance of these neurotransmitters to function properly. The most common mood-related neurotransmitters include:

Serotonin: These feel-good neuro-transmitters can control your mood, sleep patterns, and appetite. If you have low levels of serotonin, you can experience the moody blues or depression.

Epinephrine: Also known as adrenaline, this can help regulate your alertness, mental focus, and stamina. Too much stress can deplete this neurotransmitter and cause fatigue and inability to focus. High levels of epinephrine can cause anxiety, sleepless nights, and increased heart rate.

    Note: You want just the right amount.

Norepinephrine: This neurotransmitter plays an important role in your brain function and can improve your memory, mental energy, alertness, goal setting, and overall attention span.

GABA: This neurotransmitter helps calm down your body and reduce anxiety. It's a natural tranquilizer and is most effective in shutting down the body in preparation for sleep.

Dopamine: This neurotransmitter is linked to the pleasure and reward systems in the brain. It can affect your thoughts and emotions. This helps you maintain focus, think clearly, and remember things. It can also trigger addictive behavior.

Glutamate: This neurotransmitter is all about your brain development, function, and memory.

Serotonin, "ALL ABOUT THAT ZEN"

The Energy of Food

Now that we've gotten the technical stuff out of the way, let's talk about the actual foods themselves.

    Food is quite simply energy. It gives us energy to run, energy to think, and even energy to respond to trolls on Twitter (you need lots of mental stamina there!).

    It's important to recognize that every single food carries a certain energy with it. Visualize a piece of kale and a hot dog running a race. The hot dog might get off to a decent start, but that kale stalk always powers through to a sweeping first place finish.

    Every food can be placed in a specific category depending on the type of energy it carries. In Chinese medicine, this is often referred to as yin and yang—not to be confused with those black-and-white choker necklaces you wore in the '90s because you thought they were cool.

    Since our bodies are always seeking

equilibrium or balance, it's important to have a balance of energies. For example, if your body just ate kale all day long, not only would it be highly boring and void of any fun, but eventually your body would crave meatier or heartier dishes because the energy of kale would need to be balanced out. This is because kale brings a detoxifying and light energy whereas a heartier dish is more grounding and your body is attempting to balance the kale out.

Here are some of the most common food energies:

YIN AND YANG OF FOOD

In Chinese medicine, yin and yang symbolize two opposite energies that need each other to survive. If you think back to your yin–yang choker necklace or key chain, the black part represents the yin and the white part represents the yang. The dots represent the fact that there is always some yin in the yang, just as there is always some yang in the yin. So when it comes to eating, it's important to allow your body the space for both yin and yang rather than completely depriving yourself.

Foods that would be classified as yin are typically more expansive. These include sugar, coffee, alcohol, artificial chemicals and flavorings, honey, spices,

and dairy—also known as "all the good stuff." Foods low in yin include sea veggies, beans, green veggies, nuts, and seeds. All yang foods, however, are more contractive. Foods high in yang include eggs, red meat, and sea salt, and foods low in yang include grains, fish, and poultry. Yin foods typically contain a higher water content, while yang foods are dense and harder to chew.

Yin and yang foods work together to harmonize your body. For example, if you eat a diet high in sugar, which is an expansive food, you might find yourself craving salt or red meat, which are more contractive foods. Think about your own cravings. If you have something salty, you might then want something sweet. That's because your body is seeking that yin-and-yang balance.

When choosing foods and meals, it's good to have a balanced mix of yin and yang foods. For example, at breakfast time, if you are going to have some eggs, try pairing them with some greens like sautéed spinach.

Aside from their expansive and contractive qualities, yin foods tend to include more cooling foods such as juicy cantaloupes and cooling cucumbers while yang foods tend to be more warming and include foods such as garlic and ginger.

The most interesting thing about the yin and yang properties is that we, as humans, can also lean more toward yin or yang. For example, yang people are fiery and tend to be excited, full of energy, and extremely active. They are typically outgoing, outspoken, and passionate about things they care about. Yin people, on the other hand, are quieter, more grounded, and often move at a slower pace. They are often introverted and enjoy solitude. However, too much yang in a person can lead to frustration and anger whereas too much yin can lead to sadness and depression. Hence, eating an equal amount of yin and yang foods can help balance your body so that you can feel the benefits of both sides.

Aside from the physical energy properties, foods possess cooking energies as well. Raw foods are more yin, while cooked foods are more yang. That's why if you eat salads for lunch and dinner, eventually your body is going to crave something cooked and hot. Your body needs a balance of both elements.

THE ENERGY OF ANIMALS

If you choose to eat meat or if your body needs some meat, it's important to understand that each animal also has a certain energy it gives off. Think about the animal itself, what it eats, how it's raised, and understand that you take on those elements when you eat it.

For example, chickens are naturally anxious animals. Factory-farmed chickens that are forced to be in cages and pumped with feed and hormones are extremely anxious. Therefore, a diet high in chicken may eventually cause you to feel anxious.

Cows, on the other hand, are typically mellow, lethargic, and gentle. Eating *some* meat may cause you to be calm, but if you eat high quantities, you might feel slow and lethargic.

Additionally, the way animals were raised and treated and the food they ate can also carry through to our plates and into our bodies. When animals, especially factory-farmed animals, endure horrible living conditions and live in fear, the hormones released in the animals' bodies transfer into the food on our plates. The beef that might have provided grounding properties may now transfer fear-based and anxiety-inducing moods.

Meat can provide a yin-and-yang balance, but too much of it can cause emotional issues as well. When choosing meat, think about how your own body functions. If you are a naturally anxious person, too much chicken might only increase your anxiety. So skip the chicken breast and the chicken dance at cousin Susie's wedding and opt for the veggie option instead. Or maybe, if you've been on the raw food diet, your body might be craving ground beef.

It's all about finding the right type of meat for your specific body. Notice how you feel when eating a little meat compared to none at all. See how the energy of the animal provides you with energy. It's important to figure out how your body feels when eating different kinds of meat, and how much meat your body really needs.

How We Treat Food

Understanding how food has been treated before it became your dinner can also make a huge impact on your experience with that food.

When it comes to fruits and vegetables, it's important to consider whether they have been sprayed with pesticides, how long they were handled, and even how they were treated and cared for. An apple that was strictly made to look perfect and to earn the highest profits is going to give your body a different experience compared to an apple from a local family-owned orchard. These little subtleties can make all the difference in the world when it comes to our own mental health and general well-being.

Chemicals, pesticides, and added hormones used on our foods also get transferred into our digestive system and can wreak havoc. Often, we blame the food itself, when in reality, if you dig deeper, you might find that it's actually the pesticide or chemical causing your issues, not the apple or carrots.

Foods That Make You Feel Meh

Aside from satisfying cravings and providing energy, each food has various properties that can help with certain ailments, conditions, or just general well-being.

I look at the body as a super-complex machine. You can eat something one day and a week later eat the same exact thing but feel completely different. In addition to the fact that your body is always evolving, your taste buds change every six months. And you are a complex human who most likely has an existential crisis every few months.

In this section, you will learn not only what foods can make you feel like you are on top of the world but also what foods can make you feel like you are on another planet altogether.

And remember, mood-boosting foods will make you feel better physically, but it's important to pair your new eating plan with self-love and self-care, the most nutrient-dense ingredients of all.

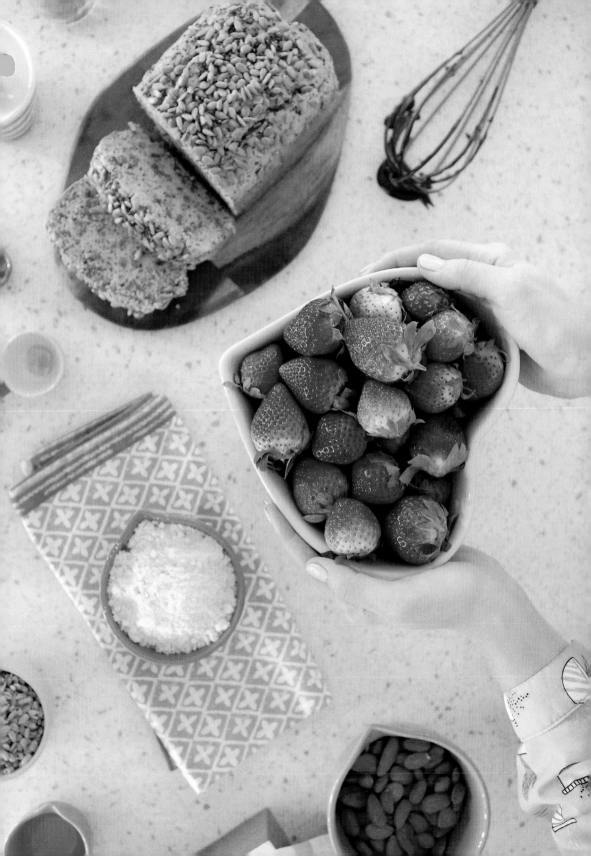

JUNK FOOD	EXAMPLES	POSSIBLE JUNK MOOD	QUICK SOLUTIONS
WHITE SUGAR	Refined sugar found in cookies, cakes, and soda; also in health food bars, organic treats	Negative mind-set, foggy thinking, fatigue, anxiety, depression	Natural sweeteners such as honey and stevia
FOOD ADDITIVES	Food dyes and colors—additives found in processed and packaged foods, even things you wouldn't expect	ADD, ADHD, negative mind-set, foggy thinking, fatigue, anxiety, depression	Juiced fruits and veggies for color and taste
CAFFEINE	Coffee, tea, chocolate	ADD, ADHD, negative mind-set, foggy thinking, fatigue, anxiety, depression, acid reflux, osteoporosis	Energizing foods like lemons, dark leafy greens, and ginger
WHITE FLOUR	Typical white breads, cookies, pastries, breading, croutons	Foggy thinking, fatigue, anxiety, depression, upset stomach	Almond flour, brown rice flour, quinoa flour, whole wheat flour

FOODS THAT DEFLATE YOUR MOOD

It's probably no surprise to anyone that junk food can greatly impact our actual mood. Junk foods can result in junk moods.

The chart above illustrates the most common energy- and mood-deflating foods. Once you know what might be deflating your mood, you can then swap it out for mood-boosting alternatives.

White Sugar

If sugar were actually sweet to our body, including our brain and our gut, as well as our mental health, then we'd be in business. White sugar is like cocaine to the brain. It gets you alert and full of energy, only to crash almost as soon as the feeling hits. We like to call this a sugar coma.

Sugar is also highly addictive. Ever wonder why you can't stop eating all the cookies even after the holiday season ends? Once we eat a little bit, sugar tricks our brain into thinking it needs

NATURAL SWEETENER	PRIMARY USES	TO REPLACE 1 CUP TABLE SUGAR	STEVIA EQUIVALENT
Agave nectar/syrup	Baking, cooking, liquids	¾ cup	¾ teaspoon
Barley malt syrup	Baking, cooking	1½ cups	1½ teaspoons
Brown rice syrup*	Baking, cooking	1½ cups	1½ teaspoons
Coconut sugar*	Baking	1 cup	1 teaspoon
Date sugar	Baking	1 cup	1 teaspoon
Honey, raw/local*	Baking, cooking, liquids	½ cup	½ teaspoon
Maple syrup*	Baking, cooking, liquids	¾ cup	¾ teaspoon
Molasses	Baking, cooking	½ cup	½ teaspoon
Stevia	Baking, cooking, liquids	1 teaspoon	———
Xylitol	Baking, cooking	1 cup	1 teaspoon
Love	Anything and everything	Unlimited!	Unlimited!

* Food Mood Girl favorites

more to extend that sweet edge and energy boost just a little longer. Sugar is hidden in almost every convenience or packaged food (organic and nonorganic alike), which makes it hard to gauge how much we are actually consuming on a daily basis.

So when it comes to white sugar, pay attention to what you are eating and how much added sugar is in it. I have found that for optimal mood benefits, eating no more than 20 grams of added sugar a day is conducive to having a healthy and clear mind, without feeling the addictive nature of sugar. But it's important to note that sugar is really where being a food-mood-etarian comes into play. Everyone has a slightly different tolerance for how much and what type of sugar they can have.

And remember, at the end of the day, even natural sweeteners are still sugar. Many of them contain extra minerals and vitamins that are good for the body, but that doesn't mean you should start thinking that a chocolate bar is equivalent to a salad (although cacao is technically a plant, so I still like to pretend it's salad from time to time).

The chart on page 35 shows some of the natural sugar alternatives you can swap into your sugary dishes. I use many of these natural sweeteners in my recipes, but feel free to experiment with new ones to discover which ones make you feel best.

Food Additives

Food additives are those pesky little ingredients added to food that tend to fly under the radar. Given that there are more than three thousand food additives approved by the FDA, it's a safe bet to say that you have most likely eaten one additive (or many) in your lifetime.

These additives, however, can react differently with everyone's bodies, and it's important to do some detective work to figure out what your body might not jibe with.

I had a client once who was sure she had a gluten/wheat allergy. However, she did all the tests and everything came back negative. She took a trip overseas and decided to indulge in some locally made bread. To her surprise, she didn't get sick.

When she came back to the United States, she figured her European vacation had healed her of her unconfirmed gluten allergy and decided to eat some bread for lunch. An hour later, she was sick. So why was the bread in Europe safe but not the bread in the United States? After some detective work, she learned that many European countries don't use food additives in their bread because it's fresh and only lasts a few days, whereas bread in the United States often has food additives in it to keep it fresh for longer. She realized that it was a food additive making her sick and not the gluten/wheat.

Since there are more than three thousand additives (and counting) in the food supply, it's often hard to pinpoint which ones are causing issues. Some of the most common food additives include:

- **Artificial colorings, such as yellow #5 and red #40:** Typically found in cereals and fruit snacks, but also can be hidden in canned foods, such as pickles, jams, condiments, and, yes, even shampoo.

- **Artificial sweeteners, such as aspartame:** Typically found in sweet foods such as cookies, cakes, and candy, and also in foods that claim to be "sugar free."

- **Monosodium glutamate:** MSG is typically found in sauces and broths. It's most common in chicken stocks, soy sauce, and foods that say they contain "natural flavorings."

- **Nitrates:** Typically found in processed meats such as hot dogs, lunch meat, ham, and sausages.

- **Partially hydrogenated vegetable oil:** Typically found in packaged foods such as chips, baked goods, and packaged snacks. It is found in margarine and coffee creamers as well.

- **Pesticides:** Typically found on nonorganic fruits and vegetables. If foods typically look perfect or are nonorganic or nonlocal, they were most likely sprayed with pesticides.

The best thing you can do for your mood and health is to limit the amount of food additives in your life by eating a minimally processed whole foods diet. However, this is real life and that won't happen all the time. So follow the steps in the box to the right when you eat something packaged or processed.

Caffeine

I still remember my first cup of coffee. Well, I guess you could say a Chocolate Brownie Frappuccino from Starbucks counts as coffee, right? I was only in eighth grade, but that little dose of caffeine was enough to send me straight

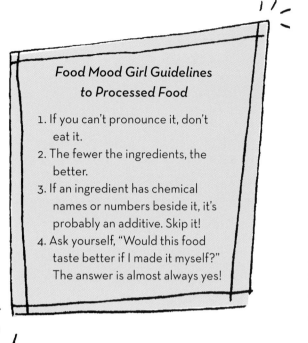

Food Mood Girl Guidelines to Processed Food

1. If you can't pronounce it, don't eat it.
2. The fewer the ingredients, the better.
3. If an ingredient has chemical names or numbers beside it, it's probably an additive. Skip it!
4. Ask yourself, "Would this food taste better if I made it myself?" The answer is almost always yes!

to becoming a java junkie. I swapped the Frappuccinos for lattes and eventually just plain black coffee.

By college, I was drinking several cups of coffee a day, using it to stay awake and alert, but eventually it stopped working. I would go for another dose at two p.m. and would still feel just as tired. I completely shot my adrenal glands from stress and anxiety, and coffee could not fix it.

So I decided to quit, cold turkey.

I had been off coffee for about five years, and for some reason, I just craved a cup. I was also curious what it would do to my body and how I would feel, so I decided to conduct a little experiment of my own.

I even made my No-Jitters Java on

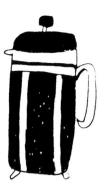

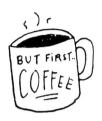

Looking for something new to try? These caffeinated and noncaffeinated beverages can help increase your energy and give you the warming sensation of coffee—and are just damn delicious: No-Jitters Java (recipe on page 209), Turmeric Tonic (page 183), and Matcha Latte (page 208).

page 209 with healthy fats and mood-boosting add-ons to give my body a sustainable boost.

Since my experiments, I've gotten to a point where I can enjoy a cup of coffee, but I don't *need* a cup of coffee.

Coffee—and caffeine specifically—is often debated among health and wellness professionals. My experiment convinced me it comes down to your own body and how you are using caffeine in your life. If you feel you are at a point where you are addicted and it's not working anymore, you might want to consider lessening your intake. Let your curiosity guide you.

From a food-and-mood standpoint, caffeine is a naturally occurring drug that can be highly addictive. Caffeine addiction can lead to increased levels of anxiety, mood swings, and sugar cravings. Stress levels can actually *increase* while you drink coffee, even though many people believe the beverage calms them down. On the flip side, coffee can help increase your alertness and improve concentration.

White Flour

Have you ever experienced the never-ending-pasta-bowl syndrome? (No, this isn't when you go to the pasta buffet and eat until you can't possibly eat any more.)

Never-ending-pasta-bowl syndrome often happens when you eat pasta, bread, a white rice dish, or something heavy with white flour. You eat and eat, but it never seems like you are getting full, so you keep eating to satisfy your hunger. Eventually you are so full that you can barely move. Then, an hour later, you find yourself hungry all over again and wonder how your stomach has suddenly become a black hole.

There is a reason for this madness that has little to do with gravity and more to do with nutrients. Foods made with white flour like white bread, pasta, crackers, and cereal, as well as white rice, are typically highly refined and stripped of nutrients. They are often referred to as "empty" because all the vitamins, minerals, and fiber are lost, never to be found again.

When you consume these empty and refined foods, your body digests them quickly since it doesn't need to spend as much time breaking down nutrients, vitamins, and fiber. It does, however, quickly convert them to sugar, giving your body a quick spike and then a sudden drop. So after eating some pasta, you feel like you can run a marathon. Then, about thirty minutes in, you'd rather be lying on your couch running through which episode of *Law & Order* you should watch first.

However, your brain isn't satisfied because it needs nutrients, not just empty calories, so it keeps searching for those nutrients by keeping you hungry. The pasta gets processed pretty quickly and then you are left looking for snacks in your cupboard and wondering why you are hungry after having downed six servings of pasta. And that is how the vicious cycle continues.

To overcome this tricky syndrome, you can start incorporating whole grains into your lifestyle. Not only are they more filling, but they also provide the nutrients your body is looking for. Whole grains are now more readily available at most grocery stores, so you no longer have to rely on brown rice for everything.

FOOD MOOD GIRL
WHITE FLOUR ALTERNATIVES

- Nut flours such as almond and cashew
- Barley
- Brown rice bread
- Brown rice flour
- Brown rice pasta (LOVE the lasagna noodles!)
- Buckwheat
- Quinoa
- Quinoa pasta
- Polenta
- Couscous
- Millet
- Rolled oats
- Wild rice
- Black rice

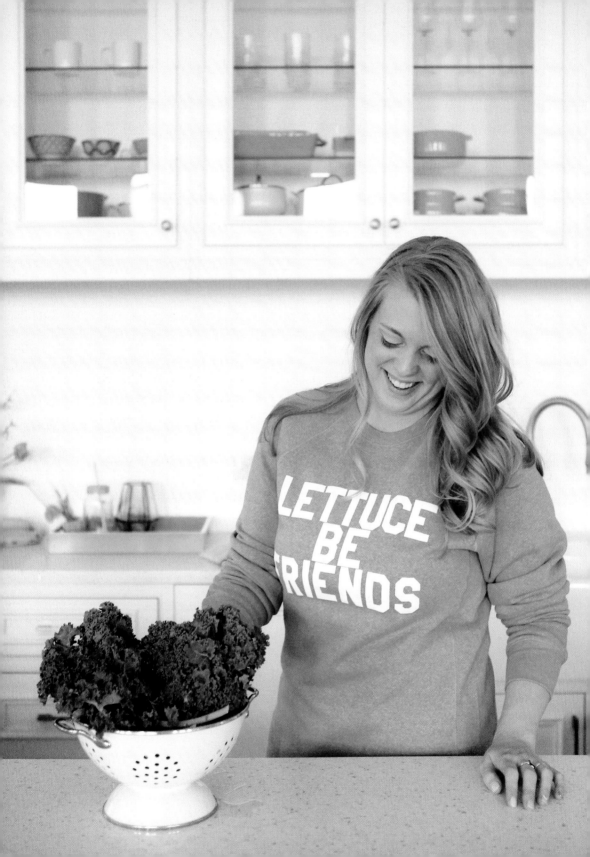

three

THE COMPLETE GUIDE TO MOOD-BOOSTING FOODS

have a big secret to share with you. It's so crazy I don't think you will be able to handle it. All fruits and vegetables have certain health benefits. I repeat, *all* fruits and vegetables serve a purpose and provide your body with certain nutrients it needs.

Sure, some are "healthier" than others, but it's important to note that most fruits, vegetables, and whole foods are mood-boosting by nature.

I remember giving a lecture about food and mood and a woman eagerly raised her hand and asked me what fruits and vegetables I thought were the best for health.

She went on and on about how she heard bananas were high in sugar and bad for you. She then went on and on about the health benefits of kale and was worried that one day she would find out it was too good to be true. I finally stopped her midway through and asked her where she was finding this information, and she quickly said, "Oh, I saw it on one of those Facebook pop-up ads."

Whoa, whoa, simmer down there! Okay, let's take a step back. First of all, stop spending so much time on Facebook and WebMD. Second of all, it's important to understand that yes, all fruits and vegetables have certain health properties. But the stress over the decision to eat kale or a banana is more detrimental to your health than just picking one and eating it.

It's tempting to look to food to solve some deep issue we have with ourselves and our bodies. We not only look at food as comfort and reward but we also imagine that a healthy food can "fix" something we don't like about ourselves. Or, even worse, we place our value in choosing what food we think is best, hoping that eventually we will match up to it. It was as if this woman thought that if I gave her a list of the top ten fruits and vegetables to eat every day, her life problems would diminish.

So even though all fruits and vegetables provide certain nutritional values and can enhance your mood and make you happier and healthier, they can't fix everything. Sometimes you have to look at those deep wounds you've been carrying around and decide you want to heal. Even on the best day, kale won't be able to heal those deep emotional cuts.

Vegetables

Artichokes: Artichokes contain more antioxidants than berries! They can help boost your immune system and prevent heart disease. They also contain the compound cynarine, which can help speed up bile production and keep your bowel movements on the regular (no coffee needed). Plus, how could you not love the fact that an artichoke has a heart?

Arugula: Known for its tangy bite, arugula is a hidden member of the cruciferous family, a group of vegetables characterized by the distinctive shape of their flowers. Arugula specifically can help lower glucose levels and combat stress.

Asparagus: Asparagus is one of the top plant-based sources of tryptophan, which your body needs to create the mood-regulating neurotransmitter serotonin. Even better, asparagus will make you feel happy because it is also high in folate, an essential vitamin known to help combat depression!

Eggplants: Eggplants can be used in dips and stews or grilled and eaten alone. However you prepare them, the amazing health benefits stay the same. Eggplants, especially the skin, contain phytonutrients that can help feed your brain. And because they're high in fiber, they can also aid healthy digestion.

Bok Choy: Typically seen in Asian cuisine, bok choy is actually a Chinese cabbage used in a variety of dishes such as soups and stir-fries. High in vitamin C, bok choy helps protect your cells against free-radical damage and helps fight off disease.

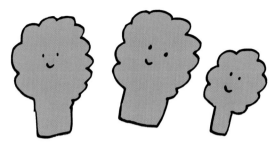

Broccoli: While these little tree-looking veggies probably first remind you of the dark times in your childhood when your parents forced you to eat your broccoli, you honestly can't blame your parents for trying. Broccoli is a cruciferous vegetable packed with vitamin C to help support your immune system, and keep your heart healthy.

Broccoli is rich in folic acid and vitamin B12, both of which appear to help prevent and alleviate mood disorders!

Brussels Sprouts: When you fed this cruciferous vegetable to your dog under the table as a kid, little did you know that you were missing out on vitamin C, vitamin K, and the nice energy boost it provides. Maybe if you filled up on the Brussels sprouts, you wouldn't have needed to eat all those Pixy Stix for your energy fix.

Cabbage: Cabbage is high in vitamin C. In fact, it has more vitamin C than an orange. So the next time you are sick or want to give your immune system a boost, try incorporating cabbage instead. Not only is it a great immune booster, but it also helps heal bleeding gums and combat depression.

Carrots: Do you prefer your carrots whole, chopped, or as sticks? Whichever way, the health benefits are the same. Carrots contain carotenoids, powerful antioxidants that help reduce free radicals in the body. Carrots also come in various shades, including orange, yellow, and purple.

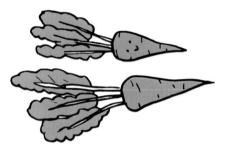

Cauliflower: This cruciferous vegetable has been making a mainstream name for itself after people realized that it does in fact taste good if cooked right, not to mention that cauliflower is high in fiber, which helps support digestion. And after all, a healthy gut equals a healthy mind.

Celery: You can do more with celery than top it with peanut butter and raisins. In fact, this water-dense vegetable is great for juicing, sautéing, and adding to soups. It also has anti-inflammatory properties, specifically in the digestive tract itself, making this a food you want to be eating when you are sad or anxious. I especially love adding celery to my Spicy Butternut Soup recipe on page 173.

Chard: Also known as Swiss chard, this powerhouse green is high in vitamin K, vitamin C, and magnesium. The combined nutrients help reduce blood pressure. Munch on some of this before an exam or presentation to help reduce your stress levels.

Collard Greens: These bone-healthy greens are high in water and fiber, which help prevent constipation—and keep you having, as the professionals call it, a regular BM. Incorporating more of these into your diet not only will give you a nice stable energy boost throughout the day, but also will help keep your hair and skin glowing.

Corn: There is truly nothing quite like fresh corn on the cob. It gives me all the summertime feelings. Aside from making you feel nostalgic, corn also provides lots of phytonutrients to help reduce disease. Eating corn really comes down to chewing it properly. Since corn contains fiber, it helps make digestion easier. But if you don't take time to fully chew it, you might just see kernels floating around your toilet bowl. (Need more on chewing? Check out page 165.)

Endive: This leafy green is typically found in your spring salad mix. It is high in manganese, which helps regulate blood sugar and maintain brain health. This is one of those foods you can eat to prevent a hangry binge later on in the day! Aside from salads, this green is an excellent add to a stir-fry or a warm pasta dish.

Kale: What the kale is going on? It seems this once-forgotten green used only to garnish plates is now a superfood champion. Truly the underdog of food, kale has proved its power to the world since it's packed with calcium, magnesium, potassium, phosphorus, and zinc. Because of the high nutrient content, leafy green vegetables are natural detoxifiers that help your body rid itself of excess toxins and leave you feeling energized. Greens are especially versatile foods. You can sauté them with garlic for a detoxifying side dish or add them to your morning smoothie for an instant energy boost.

Kohlrabi: This uncommon cabbage is a nutrient-dense powerhouse around the globe. It is used a lot in salads and slaws and has a cabbage-like consistency. It also contains more vitamin C than an orange, which can help fight off the common cold. Swap that glass of OJ for a kohlrabi slaw!

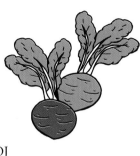

Lettuce: Like most greens, lettuce, namely butter or Bibb lettuce, can help detoxify your body and alleviate mood swings. Lettuce in particular, though, contains anxiolytic chemicals known to help reduce anxiety.

Mushrooms: Mushrooms are brain food. They contain vitamin D, boost brain function and cognition, spark serotonin receptors, and have even been shown to improve memory.

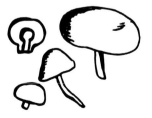

Mustard Greens: Like most other greens, mustard greens are high in vitamin K and natural detoxifiers. They are also anti-inflammatory and help protect the heart. These are perfect for stressful afternoons when your blood pressure tends to rise.

Okra: This vegetable is sometimes referred to as lady's finger, NOT to be confused with the perfected pastry known as ladyfingers. These little pods are a great source of dietary fiber and are high in mucilage, which is a substance that helps smooth digested food through the gut and prevent constipation. A gut-healthy food, okra is best served up with a rice dish or added to a stew.

Onions: Onions contain chromium, which is a natural blood regulator. They also contain sulfur, which helps lower blood sugar by triggering insulin production. Not only are they great in a variety of dishes, but these also will definitely help prevent a blood sugar crash or hangry episode.

Garlic: Garlic is part of the onion family and typically has been used for medicinal purposes throughout history. It not only smells delicious when cooking but also can help boost your immune system, kick the common cold, and reduce blood pressure.

Leeks: Leeks are closely related to the onion and garlic family, but they have a milder flavor, making them an easy add-on to soups, salads, and grain dishes. They also contain kaempferol, which is a flavonol that contains antioxidants and has anti-inflammatory properties. Leeks help alleviate low-level inflammation and stress.

Shallots: Also part of the onion family, shallots are high in flavonols, which help combat inflammation in the body. They are also high in vitamin B6, which can help calm nervous irritability. They are great sautéed, in salads, or in soups.

Chives: Chives are the smallest vegetable in the onion family and are mostly used as an herb. Chives are high in vitamin A, which is great for your eye health. Sprinkle them on a soup, salad, or baked potato as a garnish.

Peppers (green, red, bell, chili): Peppers are packed with nutritional powers. They contain vitamin C to help boost your immune system and vitamin E to help keep your skin and nails glowing. They also contain B6, which can help calm your nervous system and renew your cells. It's no wonder peppers work in almost every dish.

Radicchio: This vegetable is a perfect addition to a salad or a side dish because it's high in fiber and helps keep you fuller for longer. Say good-bye to hunger/hanger pangs! It's also high in antioxidants, which can give you an added boost of energy!

Rhubarb: This versatile vegetable is high in vitamin C, which can help give your immune system a boost, especially during the times of year when the immune system is naturally weaker. You can add rhubarb to almost anything—from pies to muffins to rice dishes to smoothies.

Beets: Beets are not only a grounding food, but they also provide your body with the extra stamina it needs to get through a busy day. They can help lower blood pressure and fight off inflammation, too. But don't forget that the bright red color of beets ends up everywhere. And I mean everywhere!

Daikon: These radishes are excellent for gut health. They contain enzymes similar to those in our digestive tract, which helps speed up digestion when we eat them. They are also

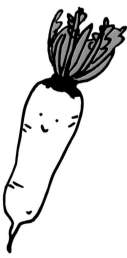

great for your skin and detoxifying your body. You can bake them, or throw them in a soup or a stir-fry. You can also eat them raw in salads or sliced up as a snack.

Ginger: Ginger is a wonder root vegetable that is known for its medicinal benefits in helping ease nausea and promote healthy digestion. It also has a great flavor in smoothies, teas, stir-fries, and curries.

Parsnips: These root vegetables are versatile in cooking and a great source of fiber and manganese. They can help boost your immune system, improve digestion, and keep your heart healthy.

Rutabaga: The rutabaga is a cruciferous vegetable that is actually a cross between a turnip and a cabbage. This is a completely gut-friendly food. It's high in fiber and help keeps you fuller for longer periods of time.

Turnips: This cruciferous vegetable is a high-fiber vegetable, which can help improve gut health and reduce inflammation in the intestinal tract. Turnips also have dietary nitrates that can help reduce blood pressure.

Spinach: If Popeye ate it and was superstrong, just imagine what it will do for you! Okay, you might not be able to lift gigantic objects after eating spinach, but it's true that spinach is great for your bone health and contains antioxidants to keep you feeling like a major boss who can take on the world. Or maybe at least conquer your afternoon meeting.

Dark leafy greens like spinach are packed with tons of vitamins, minerals, and phytochemicals that keep our brains healthy and happy. More important, though, they swiftly fight inflammation in the brain that can cause depression and sadness.

Squash: Squash comes in a variety of colors, shapes, and sizes. The most popular squashes are butternut, acorn, pumpkin, and spaghetti. However, there are dozens of squash varieties available every season. Each squash has slightly different health benefits, but for the most part, squashes are high in carotenoids and other anti-inflammatory compounds. They also promote antifungal activity and can help naturally boost your immune system. Plus, aren't they pretty to look at, reminding you of all things good about fall?

Cucumbers: Cucumbers are made up of about 95 percent water. Not only are they superhydrating, but they can also help flush out toxins. Cucumbers are also a great beauty food because they contain silica, which is a mineral that helps your hair and nails stay strong and shiny. It's truly a vegetable that beautifies you from the inside out.

WATER CONTENT = 95%

WATER CONTENT = 60%

HUMANS ARE BASICALLY CUCUMBERS wiTH ANXiETY.

Tomatoes: Pronounce it whatever way you wish, but it doesn't change the fact that this wonder fruit or vegetable (hell, I still don't know!) is high in antioxidants, which can help combat oxidative stress in the bones and reduce the risk of heart disease. There are hundreds of varieties of tomatoes to choose from, depending on your taste. Tomato skin contains lycopene, a fat-soluble phytonutrient that protects brain fat and actually combats the types of inflammation linked to depression.

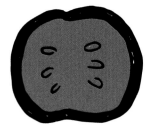

Zucchini: While zucchini is technically a fruit (I know, I was shocked to learn this myself!), it is prepared like a vegetable. You can eat it raw, grilled, sautéed, or baked. Zucchini is high in manganese and vitamin C, which can help prevent bruising and keep your joints operating smoothly.

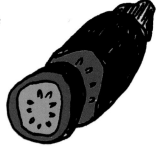

Sweet Potatoes: Characterized by their bright orange hue, sweet potatoes are high in antioxidants and also help regulate blood sugar levels. They also are sweet and versatile to cook with. You can make mashed sweet potatoes, grilled sweet potatoes, sweet potato pie, or simply enjoy a baked sweet potato.

Potatoes: Mashed, roasted, baked, or in the form of French fries, potatoes are a longtime staple as they are available year-round and come in a wide variety. Potatoes contain high levels of vitamin B6 and potassium, which can help the nervous system, especially the brain, and provide heart support.

Tatsoi: These powerhouse greens are full of phytochemicals and calcium. Believe it or not, a single serving of fresh tatsoi leaves has more calcium than a glass of milk. They are typically found in Asian cuisine and are great in stir-fries and salads. While these greens have a unique name, they are actually very common and can often be found in greens mixes at local farmers' markets or Asian grocery stores.

Watercress: This cruciferous plant is an underrated wonder plant. It contains folate, which can help combat depression, as well as high levels of vitamin C (seriously, more than an orange!), which can help your immune system and brain. You can use watercress like any other green: in salads, soups, pastas, casseroles, sauces, or smoothies!

Fruits

Apples: There are more than a hundred varieties of apples to choose from, and they all contain phytonutrients that help prevent hypertension, diabetes, and heart disease. Apples also contain fiber, which keeps your digestion regular.

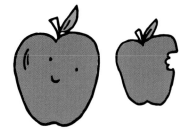

Apricots: These tiny but mighty fruits are packed with vitamin A, potassium, and fiber. They have high amounts of soluble fiber, which helps promote a healthy glucose level and keep cholesterol levels down.

Avocados: Is it just me, or did avocados suddenly become the new black? These high-fat fruits (yes, avocados are fruits!) are amazing at giving your brain a boost and keeping you fuller for longer. They are smooth and creamy and can be used in sweet or savory dishes. They also contain more potassium than bananas, which helps regulate blood pressure. And lastly, this powerhouse of a fruit also helps you absorb more antioxidants in other foods that you eat. Many foods are fat-soluble, meaning that to get the most nutrients possible, you need to eat them with fat. Since avocados feature a healthy fat, they can extract the most antioxidants with every bite.

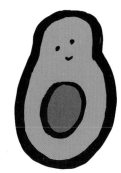

Bananas: This sweet "fast food" not only is one of the most popular fruits but also is high in fiber, helping digestion. Bananas also contain high amounts of pectin, a resistant starch, which can help keep you fuller for longer. This can help reduce cravings and keep you from overeating. And since bananas are naturally sweet, you can substitute them for sugar in many baked goods.

Blackberries: Similar to other berries, blackberries are high in antioxidants, which can help lower the risk of cancer, boost the immune system, and preserve your skin's youthful glow. Additionally, they give your brain a boost by maintaining mental clarity.

Blueberries: Aside from the high levels of vitamin C that help combat stress, blueberries are also full of antioxidants, specifically anthocyanin, which improves brain function.

Cherries: Cherries contain melatonin, which is a powerful antioxidant and natural sleep supporter. Additionally, cherries are anti-inflammatory and can help relieve joint pain. Tart cherry juice provides the antioxidant power of cherries in a concentrate.

Coconuts: When you're stressed out, coconut can act fast to soothe you by physically slowing your heart rate and reducing blood pressure. Amazingly, coconut has been shown to enhance alertness while simultaneously soothing stress.

Cranberries: Cranberries can help lower the risk of urinary tract infections. Additionally, they help support immune function and decrease blood pressure. And believe it or not, concentrated cranberry juice can help prevent gum disease and whiten teeth over time!

Dates: If you've got a sweet tooth but want to stay happy and healthy, try some dates. Their rich texture and sweet taste will leave you satisfied, but unlike candy, dates are full of fiber, vitamins, minerals, and antioxidants to keep your energy up.

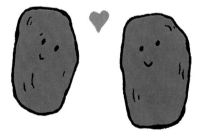

Elderberries: Elderberry is a major immune system booster, alleviating coughs, colds, and various infections. It is also high in fiber, which can increase the nutrients you absorb in your gut so you get the most bang for your buck when eating whole foods.

Figs: When I think of figs, the first thing I think of is the Fig Newton cookies I used to eat as a kid. But these delicious fruits can help boost the immune system and combat respiratory issues. Since they are low in sodium and high in potassium, they are known as a calming food and can help settle tension and nerves.

Grapes: Do you like green, purple, or red grapes? Seedless or full of seeds? There are so many options, but the health benefits are the same. Grapes are high in antioxidants and have been shown to help resolve skin issues. They also contain quercetin, which is a flavonoid that helps to naturally lower cholesterol. Regardless of how you eat (or drink) these fruits, always remind yourself that "you're grape."

Raisins: Raisins are dehydrated grapes that actually become more nutritionally concentrated. They are also high in iron and can help keep your brain sharp and your energy levels high. Additionally, they contain phytonutrients that can combat fevers and viral infections. They are great to mix into a salad or eat as a midday snack on their own.

Grapefruit: High in vitamin C, this fruit helps boost your immune system and keep you healthy all year round. It's also high in water content, which can help flush out fat and toxins as well as make you feel full and hydrated. Just the smell of this citrus fruit is enough to curb stress, anxiety, and depression. It's also great in a salad.

Guava: This wonder fruit is anti-inflammatory and antibacterial, which means it can help alleviate joint pain and fight off infections. Additionally, it contains high amounts of magnesium, which can combat physical stress and help nerves in the body relax.

Huckleberries: No, I don't mean Huckleberry Finn. I mean the actual berry. Similar to most berries, huckleberries contain antioxidants that can help fight free radicals and improve the quality of your skin.

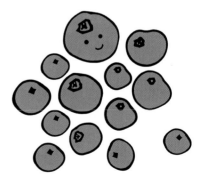

Jackfruit: Often known as the "jack of all fruits" because it is high in B vitamins, vitamin C, vitamin A, and fiber, the jackfruit also contains electrolytes to keep the body refreshed and can be used in a variety of ways. It looks a little bit scary on the outside, but it has a sweet and delicious interior that is ready to give your body a boost. It's also great to use as a vegan substitute for meat. You can flavor it with your favorite spices and bake or sauté it to create tacos or meaty sandwiches.

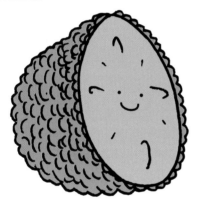

Kiwis: These small but mighty fruits are packed with vitamin C, helping boost immunity and keep your skin clear. And if you are having trouble falling asleep at night, kiwis have been shown to help you get your *z*'s by limiting sleep disturbances.

Kumquats: If you need a quick yet sustainable energy boost, this little fruit will do the trick. It's also high in fiber and water, which can help eliminate toxins and beat bloating.

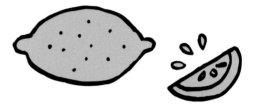

Lemons: Lemons have amazing benefits for the entire body. Even though they are acidic in their natural state, combined with the body's natural fluids, they actually help alkalinize the body and balance pH levels. They are also stimulating to the entire body. Not only will they get your mind and brain going, but they will get your digestion going, too. Check out the Iced Turmeric Lemonade on page 183 to set up your day for success!

Limes: Got bad BO? Grab a lime and put it on your pits. Just please don't do this in a grocery store as you might get asked to leave. But seriously, limes contain a high amount of vitamin C and can help keep your hair shiny, your skin clear, and your pits from smelling like a hoagie. (Come on, you know they smell like Subway after an intense workout.) Limes also help regulate blood sugar to keep your mood stable all day long.

Mangoes: Not only are mangoes a sweet treat to eat, but they also can be used externally as a nourishing face mask. Eating mangoes or applying mango masks can help reduce inflammation and breakouts on the skin. They also have a low glycemic index, so they won't spike your blood sugar like other fruits.

Cantaloupe: A popular summer fruit, cantaloupe helps combat the heat and hydrate your body. It's high in potassium, which can help decrease blood pressure and calm physical stress. It's also high in vitamin C, which makes it a great food for your skin, hair, and nails. It's another fruit that you can eat or apply directly to your hair to add moisture and shine.

Honeydew: This sweet fruit is another hydrating fruit that can combat dehydration and detoxify the body. It's also high in vitamin C, which regulates collagen, helping nourish skin tissue and blood vessels. This leads to a healthy and happy glow.

Mulberries: These sweet berries are typically found in jams and teas, but fresh mulberries contain high amounts of iron, resveratrol, and carotenoids. These nutrients can help combat oxidative stress, reduce the chance of heart issues, and speed up metabolism.

Nectarines: This fruit can help you digest carbohydrates, which makes it a gut-friendly food. It also contains potassium, which can boost metabolism and regulate pH balance.

Olives: Whether you love 'em or hate 'em, these small but mighty fruits are jam-packed with benefits. They are a great source of iron, which is helpful if you are feeling sluggish or low-energy. Pop a couple of olives for a quick energy boost. They are an anti-inflammatory food as well, and they can reduce your chance of head pain. They also help produce higher levels of serotonin in the blood, which makes you feel fuller for longer and gives you that "I can do anything" feeling.

Oranges: Oranges contain vitamin C, which has been shown to help lower blood pressure and cortisol levels, making this fruit the ultimate stress reliever. Just the smell of oranges can bring a sense of joy, energy, and happiness. So whether you are eating one or you simply get a whiff of one, you are getting some healthy benefits for your body and mind.

Clementines: These are the ultimate brain food! Clementines contain folate, which can help the brain function properly, reducing stress, anxiety, and depression. They also contain fiber, which helps relax digestive muscles, making it easier to keep a healthy tract. Plus, they are supercute—and that alone just makes you smile.

Mandarins: Mandarins, just like their cousin the orange, contain large amounts of vitamins A, B, and C, which can help boost the immune system, regulate blood pressure, and give you a healthy glow. The best part is this little fruit can be tossed in a salad to give it a sweet taste or eaten whole as a snack.

Papaya: This gut-friendly fruit contains papain, which helps digestion, and can be used to tenderize meat to make it easily digestible, too. It also contains fiber and a high water content, helping you keep those bowel movements regular.

Passion Fruit: This pretty fruit is a natural mood booster and sleep inducer. It contains alkaloids, which are phytonutrients known for their sedative tendencies, helping ease the nervous system and combat issues such as anxiety,

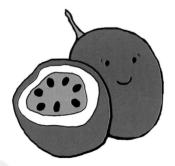

depression, and insomnia. This calming fruit is excellent juiced and can help reduce stress symptoms in just a few sips.

Peaches: These fuzzy fruits aren't just for pies! Peaches in their natural state make a great snack and can help keep you full. Additionally, they contain phytonutrients that can help calm nerves and reduce anxiety. They also help calm upset stomachs with those same properties. In Hungary, peaches are known as the "fruit of calmness." And hey, if it's in a pie, I guess that doesn't hurt either!

Pears: These smooth fruits are one of the highest in fiber, which can help beat belly bloat and keep your digestive tract operating smoothly. They're also a hypoallergenic fruit, which is helpful for people who have a lot of food sensitivities. Plus, they are underrated and taste delicious in salads, on sandwiches, or by themselves.

Persimmon: Is that an orange tomato? Nope, it's a persimmon. These tasty fruits contain a ton of antioxidants, which can help boost your immune system and reduce your sick day usage. They also contain high levels of vitamin C and potassium. This can help regulate blood pressure and relax muscles, making it the perfect snack to help your body relax.

Plantains: This banana look-alike provides health benefits of its own. It's high in potassium and fiber, which can help regulate blood pressure and the digestive tract. It also contains magnesium, which can help prevent headaches, insomnia, and depression. Plantains aren't as sweet as bananas, but they are great grilled, fried, or even prepared as chips.

Plums: Plums can help keep your heart healthy and your blood sugar levels stable. They are also a mental-health-enhancing food, containing powerful antioxidants that can help improve your memory and keep your brain sharp. These make a great pretest snack to ensure you are alert and focused.

Prunes (dried plums): Does Granny have any prune juice in her fridge? While the juice may be considered an "old person" drink, prunes are a great source of energy without the blood sugar crash that other foods give you. And yes, prunes are high in fiber, which can help keep you regular. But let's face it, everyone can benefit from that, not just Granny!

Pineapples: Pineapples contain bromelain, which is an enzyme that can help reduce inflammation, especially in the sinuses. And if you need a quick energy boost, pineapples contain

manganese and thiamine, which help your body produce energy. And if you still don't know how to cut a damn pineapple, check out page 95.

Pomegranates: Pomegranates not only make a delicious juice, but the seeds also can be sprinkled on salads, proteins, or even on baked dishes like Brussels sprouts. They contain polyphenols, which can help your gums and prevent plaque, and antioxidants that can help reduce inflammation and lower blood pressure. Check out the Made-with-Love Brussels recipe with pomegranate on page 197.

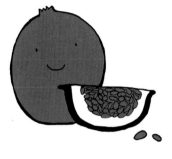

Raspberries: These tiny berries contain carotenoids and citric acid, which can help reduce muscle cramps, tension, and stress. They also help reduce inflammation and pain throughout the body. Pop a few raspberries in your mouth, sit back, and relax.

Strawberries: Remember when your parents would soak your strawberries in sugar water and feed them to you as a "healthy snack"? Or was this just my family? Either way, strawberries in their natural form have a low glycemic index and are filled with antioxidants and chock-full of vitamin C. They help fight off free radicals and support your immune system.

Watermelon: The most popular summer fruit not only is fun to eat but also contains a bunch of nutrients to keep your mood, joints, and body healthy. This sweet fruit contains lycopene, antioxidants, and amino acids. It is especially high in vitamins A and C, and has been shown to help reduce blood pressure—in other words, keeping you calm during a meltdown.

Mood-Boosting Extras

For a long time, I was always adding weird and hard-to-find "superfoods" to my baked goods, smoothies, and sautés. These superfoods are nutrient-rich and tend to have higher amounts of certain vitamins and minerals that are beneficial to health and well-being. While I love them, I also understand that having a shelf full of once-opened $20 packages of weird add-ins whose names you can't pronounce is probably not doing your mood or your bank account any good.

It also sucks when someone online posts a recipe called something like "The Natural Non-Acidic Coffee You Need in Your Life" and you are so excited to check it out. Then you click on it only to find that the recipe includes like twenty weird superfoods, only a half teaspoon of each, and it will cost you about $160 to attempt to make a drink you may or may not like.

My theory on superfoods is that they can be used as a mood-boosting extra in meals, but it's important to be realistic with yourself. Maybe try one at a time to see how you like it and how you can incorporate it. Or even shop the bulk section at your local natural food store and try a little bit of something to see if you like it first. Sure, these foods have lots of benefits, but you will get those benefits only if you actually like and use them, so purchase wisely!

Most of the superfoods listed here can now be found at most conventional grocery stores. Surprisingly, stores like T.J. Maxx and Marshalls also have a wide selection of superfoods available. And if all else fails, there is Amazon.

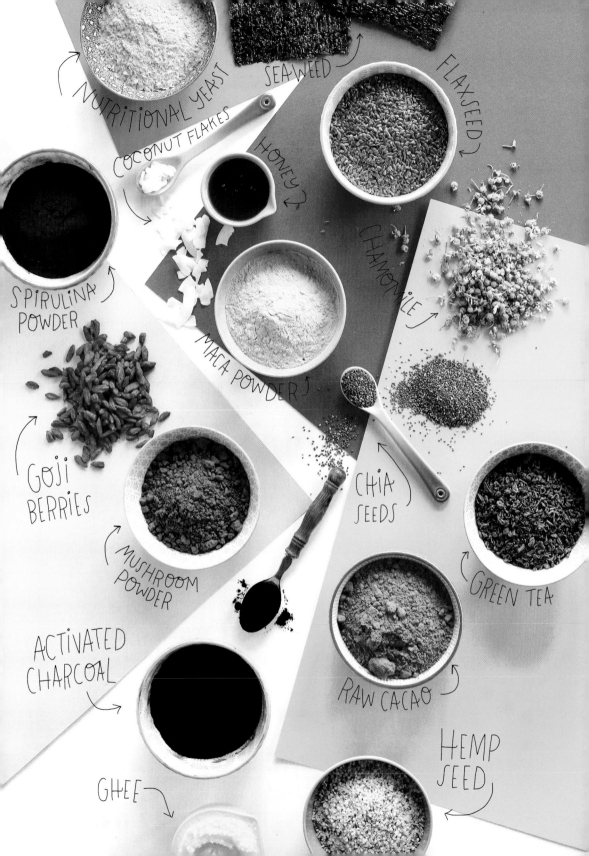

NUTRITIONAL YEAST

SEAWEED

FLAXSEED

COCONUT FLAKES

HONEY

CHAMOMILE

SPIRULINA POWDER

MACA POWDER

GOJI BERRIES

CHIA SEEDS

MUSHROOM POWDER

GREEN TEA

ACTIVATED CHARCOAL

RAW CACAO

HEMP SEED

GHEE

Here are some of my favorite mood-boosting extras:

Chia Seeds: Ch-ch-ch-chia! Remember those little fuzzy-headed Chia Pets? You could get them in cute animals and not-so-cute presidents. Chia seeds are the magic trick behind those infomercial plants. Don't let the Chia Pet fool you, though, because actual chia seeds are great for your mood. These little seeds are packed with nutrients, high in fiber, and a great source of omega-3 fatty acids. And while they won't actually sprout in your stomach, they will expand slightly, making you feel full, so you will be less likely to overeat.

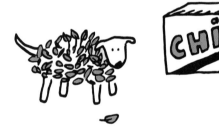

Raw Cacao: Pronounced *cuh-cow*. Unlike store-bought cocoa powder, raw cacao contains nutrients that give your body and brain a boost. Cacao is high in antioxidants, iron, magnesium, chromium, manganese, and zinc. It's also rich in tryptophan, which is used to produce serotonin, helping boost your mood, alleviate brain fog, and reduce anxiety. When eating cacao, phenyl ethylamine is also released, which can have the same effect on your brain and body as falling in love. So here's a good trick: give your significant other some raw cacao powder for Valentine's Day and really spice things up. Or just use some year-round for mood-enhancing goodness.

Spirulina: This green powder is derived from algae—not the kind on your childhood fish tank that you were always too grossed out to clean, but algae that grows in mineral-rich and pollution-free lakes around the world. It's high in protein, chlorophyll, and iron, which can help boost your energy and reduce brain fog. I personally like adding spirulina to my smoothies—and just a little bit goes a long way.

Coconut Oil: I got ninety-nine problems and coconut oil can fix all of them. Seriously, coconut oil is the food of the century. It's high in he good kind of saturated fat and can be used in cooking or baking. It is especially useful for high-heat cooking. The healthy fat helps support your brain, your nervous system, and your skin. Aside from eating coconut oil, you also can use it topically on your skin or even mixed with essential oils

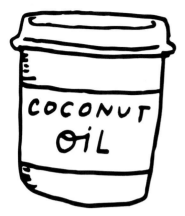

Maca Powder: This potent powder from a Peruvian root is an amazing mood booster and hormone balancer. It is rich in magnesium, calcium, phosphorus, potassium, iron, and B vitamins, making it a superfood that can help with everything from relieving PMS symptoms to increasing energy.

Goji Berries: Goji berries are a complete source of protein and contain all the essential amino acids, helping keep you full, satisfied, and calm. They are perfect to put on salads, in trail mix, in smoothies, or even in your favorite dessert. The sweet and tangy flavor goes well with just about anything.

such as peppermint or tea tree oil to make a teeth whitener.

Flaxseeds: These small seeds are one of the highest sources of omega-3 fatty acids outside of fish. The high levels of omega-3 fatty acids help keep energy high and the brain and immune system functioning properly. These can be mixed in a smoothie or in baked goods. You can even use flaxseeds as an egg substitute if you want to make a dish vegan or egg-free.

Seaweed: Seaweed is a superfood to be reckoned with. You've most likely seen seaweed, known as *nori* in Japanese, in sushi rolls. However, now you also can find kelp flakes to sprinkle on fries, salads, soups, and other dishes, as well as seaweed snacks that can be eaten on the go. Seaweed contains folic acid, which helps make serotonin and can lift depression and give your mood a boost. Seaweed is naturally salty, which can help curb your salt cravings and give your body the minerals it needs.

Hemp Seeds: These little seeds won't get you high, but they will give you a nice brain boost. They are complete proteins that are high in phosphorus, magnesium, potassium, manganese, and iron. They are also rich in omega-3 fatty acids, which support brain function and memory. Sprinkle these on a soup or salad for an extra crunch and some added protein.

Nutritional Yeast: Often we hear the word "yeast" and think we either are baking bread or have an infection. But nutritional yeast is not an active yeast, which means that it has no effect on the body besides passing on the general health benefits of yeast. It's jam-packed with B vitamins, folic acid, selenium, and zinc. It's also antiviral and antibacterial, qualities that allow it to help fight off infections and keep your body moving. You can sprinkle it on salads, add it to soups, or use it to help create creaminess in nondairy dishes.

Wheatgrass: Consuming just two ounces of this potent grass is like eating five pounds of fruits and vegetables. Wheatgrass contains all the essential minerals to keep your body going and is especially rich in protein and amino acids. It also can help improve digestion and balance blood sugar, two crucial things to keep your mood and spirits high.

Raw or Local Honey: Most store-bought honey contains high-fructose corn syrup. (Bummer, right?!) Getting your honey raw or from local providers is the best way to ensure quality and taste. It's a great substitute for sugar because it is packed with nutrients your body needs such as amino acids, enzymes, and minerals like iron, magnesium, potassium, and zinc. Additionally, local honey can help people who suffer from bee-sting allergies experience fewer symptoms as they are ingesting local pollen, which can help build immunity to it.

A few ways to check if your honey is real:

1. The only ingredient on the label should be honey. (Depending on what ingredients the food manufacturers used, they might not have to list all the ingredients on the back, though, which means it could still be fake.)
2. True honey is pretty thick and will take a while to move from one side of a jar to the other. Fake honey, on the other hand, is thin, runny, and light.
3. Real honey might have some impurities in it like pollen or honeycomb particles, whereas fake honey will be almost perfectly clear and consistent.

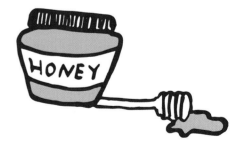

Chaga or Reishi Mushroom Powder: Chaga and reishi mushrooms have typically been used in teas. These powerful mushrooms have a wide range of health benefits, including boosting the immune system, alleviating joint pain, balancing blood sugar, and protecting cells. They've been known to fight stress and are a natural energy booster. The powder makes a great addition to soups or hot drinks.

Saffron: This tasty spice has been shown to be a natural antidepressant, strong enough to have its effects compared clinically to Prozac!

Vanilla: Vanilla offers an abundance of health benefits, including being a good source of potassium, calcium, and manganese, but just the scent of vanilla has been proven to trigger happy, relaxed, and even sensuous feelings. So grab a vanilla latte and inhale a big whiff while sipping!

Turmeric: Turmeric has anti-inflammatory properties and has also been found to function like an antidepressant. And curcumin, turmeric's active ingredient, enhances nerve growth in the brain.

Spicy Ginger Root Powder: Not to be confused with the hair color or the Spice Girl, ginger root is a powerful antioxidant that helps combat digestive issues and nausea. Ginger is also an anti-inflammatory food, helping to alleviate joint pain and muscle soreness. It can help lower blood sugar and keep your moods stabilized as well.

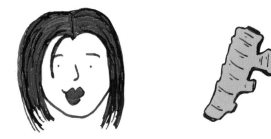

Green Tea: This type of tea is a powerful antioxidant that can help improve concentration, relieve anxiety, and boost energy. While the most common way of consuming green tea is by brewing a cup, you also can add a bag or two to boiling rice, pasta, or other grains while they are cooking. The grains will absorb the powerful antioxidants the green tea has to offer, and you will give your dish an additional mood boost without much extra effort.

Chamomile: This wonder flower helps reduce anxiety and promote a calm mental attitude with its powerful flavonoids. Drink a cup of chamomile tea

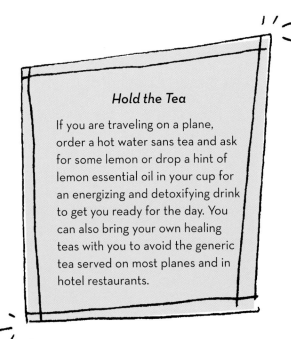

sweet, adding honey or maple syrup, raisins, and cinnamon. Or you can even make it savory and add some pesto, sun-dried tomatoes, and an egg. Oatmeal contains high levels of selenium, a mineral that acts like an antioxidant in the body and relieves oxidative stress on the brain, alleviating symptoms of depression and seasonal affective disorder. Oatmeal is especially good to eat in the winter months since it's both warming and combative of the wintertime blues.

Quinoa: Pronounced *keen-wah*. Quinoa is considered the queen of the grains. Well, not officially by any sort of fancy organization, but there is reason for my declaration. Quinoa is one of the most nutrient-dense foods available and the only grain that contains all the essential amino acids, making it a complete plant-based protein. Aside from its high nutritional profile, quinoa is also gluten-free and easy to digest. It can be served cold with chopped vegetables and dressing for a simple and refreshing salad, or it can be warmed with spices like cinnamon for an energizing and delicious breakfast.

before bed to help relax and wind down after a busy day.

Ghee: Ghee is clarified butter, cooked down to remove the water and milk, turning it into a high-smoke-point oil. You can use ghee as cooking oil or spread it on a piece of toast. Since ghee is fat-soluble, it helps your body naturally absorb fat-soluble vitamins such as A, D, and E. Increasing vitamin D can help alleviate seasonal affective disorder.

Grains

Oatmeal: There are so many delicious ways to eat oatmeal. You can make it

Millet: This gluten-free grain is less common than rice or quinoa but contains similar health benefits. Millet can help keep the digestive track moving, increase

bran, which makes it more nutrient-dense. While each rice variant has different nutritional properties, rice in general is easy to digest, gluten-free, and full of antioxidants. Rice can also help stabilize blood sugar levels, preventing the crash that empty carbohydrates often leave the body with.

Couscous: While technically couscous resides in the pasta family, it can be used in recipes wherever grains are used and takes only five minutes to make. This is great for a quick and easy side dish, while still giving you your protein, fiber, and B vitamins. It can be eaten hot or cold and used as a substitute in most grain recipes. When you are hangry, simply cook up some couscous and combine it with some salsa for a quick and easy snack.

energy, and detoxify the body. It makes a great breakfast porridge in lieu of oatmeal or can be a part of a main dish, side, or snack. Check out the Cauliflower Burger on page 223 to try millet. Make a little extra to try it for breakfast porridge the next day, too!

Barley: Barley is another less-common grain. It's actually one of the oldest grains, with substantial health benefits. Barley has fewer calories and more fiber than most other grains on the market, making it a filling and digestion-friendly food. Barley is also high in selenium, which can help combat oxidative stress and keep you feeling calm. You can eat barley as a side dish, mixed in a hot bake or a cold salad, or even in cookies and snacks.

Rice: Wild rice, black rice, and brown rice contain the grain's original hull and

Nuts and Seeds

Most nuts and seeds are high in fiber, protein, and healthy fats. The healthy-fat-and-protein combination helps keep your brain functioning so you don't start every sentence in the middle of the workday with "Um, I forget what I was going to say." Additionally, the fiber intake keeps you full of energy. Combined with the powerful concentration, you will be able to move through your day accomplishing

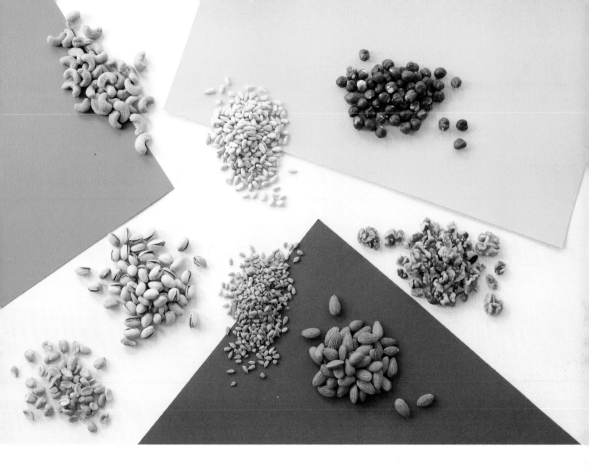

tasks at record speed. Also: pecan pie, while delicious, will not have the same side effects that whole nuts and seeds have.

Some staples include:

- Almonds
- Brazil nuts
- Cashews: These little nuts are a great source of zinc, which is shown to naturally reduce anxiety.
- Chia seeds
- Flaxseeds
- Hazelnuts
- Macadamia nuts
- Peanuts (technically a legume, but often known as a nut)
- Pecans
- Pine nuts
- Pistachios
- Pumpkin seeds: Pumpkin seeds are rich in magnesium, an essential mineral that protects you from anxiety and depression. More than that, pumpkin seeds are a good source of zinc and omega-3 fatty acids. Feeling restless? The tryptophan in pumpkin seeds can also help you catch up on some sleep!

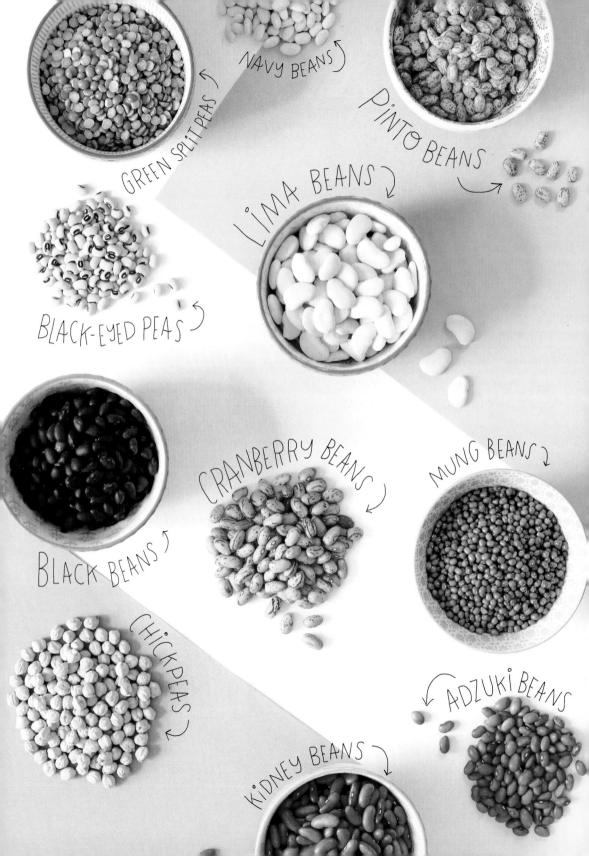

GREEN SPLIT PEAS ↱

NAVY BEANS ↰

PINTO BEANS →

LIMA BEANS ↓

BLACK-EYED PEAS ↱

CRANBERRY BEANS ↴

MUNG BEANS ↰

BLACK BEANS ↰

↙ ADZUKI BEANS

CHICKPEAS ↴

KIDNEY BEANS ↓

- Sesame seeds
- Sunflower seeds
- Walnuts: Because our brains are 80 percent fat, we need healthy fats to sustain their function. Enter walnuts. These supernuts keep your brain fed with a steady dose of omega-3s, keeping you happy and energized all day long!

Beans and Legumes

Most beans and legumes are packed with protein and have a low glycemic index, which means that your body digests them slowly, keeping your blood sugar stable so you avoid energy crashes or hanger

Food Mood Girl Love Note

Foods that are sprouted typically have a higher nutritional value because they contain more enzymes compared to uncooked fruits and vegetables. These enzymes can improve your gut health and your immune system. And the best part? You can sprout your own at home. Simply put some alfalfa sprouts in a jar, watch them sprout, and add them to smoothies, sandwiches, salads, and sautés.

episodes. They are also packed with fiber, which will help keep your digestive track flowing regularly and keep you feeling fuller longer so your chances of eating out of boredom decrease. And with the many varieties of beans and legumes, from dry to fresh to canned, they are accessible, inexpensive, and extremely versatile when cooking.

Some staples include:

- Adzuki beans
- Alfalfa sprouts
- Bean sprouts
- Black beans
- Black-eyed peas
- Chickpeas
- Chili beans
- Cranberry beans
- Green beans
- Green split peas
- Kidney beans
- Lentils
- Lima beans
- Mung beans
- Navy beans
- Pinto beans
- Snow peas
- Sugar snap peas

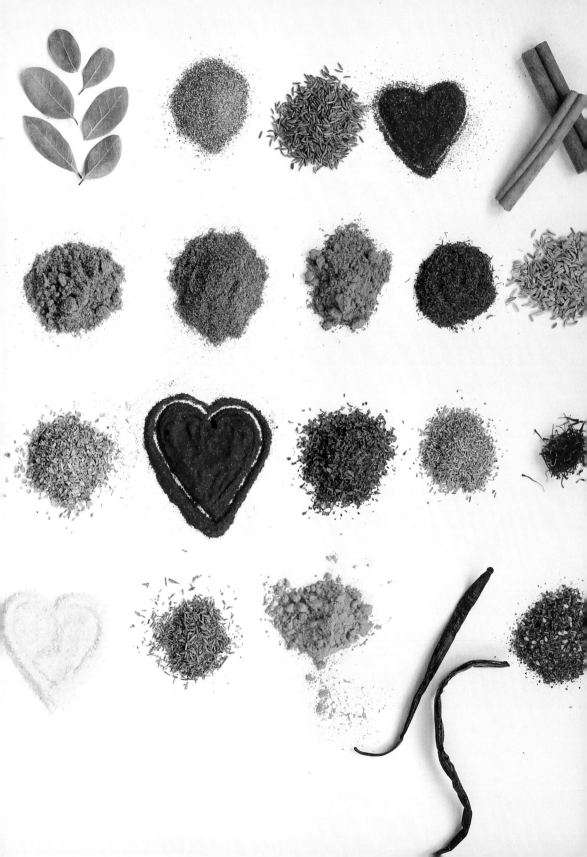

Herbs and Spices

I call herbs and spices the "mood enhancers" because not only do they add flavor, but many of them provide additional health benefits as well. They can help expand your food's flavor profile without extra salt, fat, or sugar. Herbs and spices also help flavor your food so you feel satisfied. Many times bland foods can leave us feeling empty and wanting more because we are searching for a certain flavor that we are not getting.

Some staples include:

- Basil
- Caraway
- Chamomile
- Cilantro
- Curry powder
- Dill
- Fennel seeds
- Lavender
- Lemongrass
- Oregano
- Parsley
- Rosemary
- Sage
- Sumac
- Thyme
- Za'atar

I CALL HERBS AND SPICES THE "MOOD ENHANCERS..."

Lazy Susan

A lazy Susan is a round turntable tray that is often used in the kitchen for organization. My favorite way to use it is with spices and condiments. Oftentimes, I'll create dishes and encourage my guests to flavor them with various spices and flavors. The lazy Susan makes spices accessible and easy to use. Since people have different palates, this ensures that everyone can enjoy their favorite flavors.

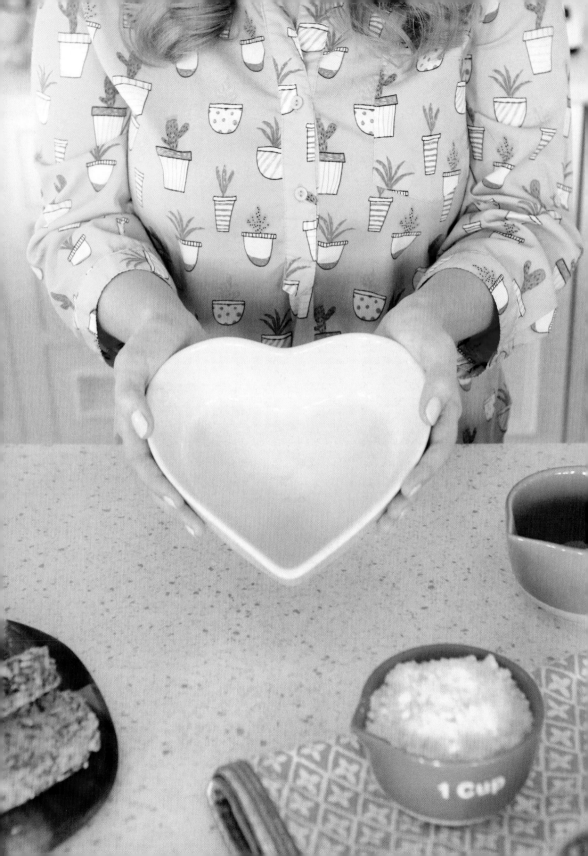

four

FOOD MOOD PANTRY MAKEOVER

When people hear the phrase "pantry makeover," their initial instinct is to throw away everything deemed "bad" for you and fill it up with "good" food. However, that can actually end up causing more issues down the line, including food guilt, food waste, and a never-ending cycle of buying bad shit, throwing it away, and replacing it with stuff you have no idea what the hell to do with.

So first, don't throw out everything you own, unless, of course, it's expired and growing mold. Then yes, for everyone's sake, throw it out! (Or compost it!)

Once you do that, follow these simple steps to change the way you think about food and your pantry.

1. **Swap, Don't Toss:** Once you finish an item, try swapping it for a healthier alternative the next time you shop. For example, if you love Fruit Roll-Ups, try swapping it for fruit leather or dried fruit instead. Do this little by little until you create a new way of living.
2. **Shop Often:** Next consider the way in which you shop. Most busy people tend to have one big grocery day of the week, buy enough food to last two weeks, and waste half of it by the time the next week rolls around. I, too, wish that fresh vegetables had the shelf life of a bag of Oreos, but unfortunately they

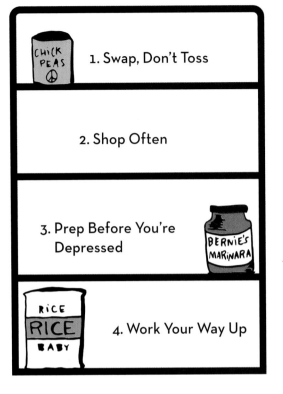

1. Swap, Don't Toss

2. Shop Often

3. Prep Before You're Depressed

4. Work Your Way Up

don't. However, if you shop every few days for the things you are making every few days, you will end up wasting less and feeling more fulfilled in the long run. The best thing you can do for yourself, your health, and the planet is to buy fresh produce a few days before you make it. It takes some getting used to, but it will eventually save you time and money down the road.

3. **Prep Before You're Depressed:** If you know that you have a big work event happening that will most likely zap your energy, then prep food the day before so that you have your ingredients ready to go for an easy dinner creation. While you can't always control what happens or how you feel throughout the day, you can notice patterns or things that affect you and can therefore try to prep before you're feeling down. You can also prep some freezer meals ahead of time to reheat or throw in the slow cooker for those unexpected mood-sucking days.

4. **Work Your Way Up:** The most important thing you can do is work your way up to creating a healthy fridge and pantry. As stated earlier, the last thing you want to do is throw away everything you've ever bought and replace it with stuff you don't even know what to do with. This will leave you irritated and most likely hangry when you can't figure out what to make. Allow this process to be ongoing and to evolve as you embark on your journey.

The Fridge Scene: Creating a Healthy and Mood-Friendly Fridge

FRESH FRUITS AND VEGGIES

Let's get one thing straight: fruits and vegetables are amazing. Seriously, every

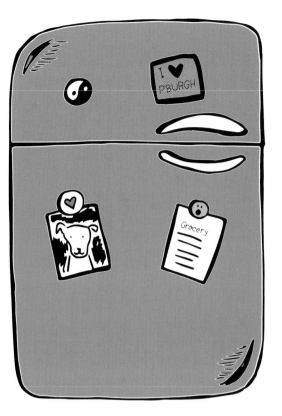

with the food mood mapping guide in chapter 5. As you start to become more aware of your body, you will recognize what foods work for your unique body.

- **Local and seasonal is best.** Don't get me wrong—sometimes I want mangoes in the middle of winter and I won't stop until I get them. But eating as closely as you can to your local and seasonable climate is best. This is because foods in season and grown locally are typically meant to help assist your body through the changing season.
- **Be open to trying something new.** My rule of thumb is to try one new fruit or vegetable I've never seen before or tried anytime I go grocery shopping or stop at the farmers' market. Even things we never liked as kids, we can grow to enjoy as adults. Your taste buds are always changing (every six months, to be exact), so be open to treating your palate to something new. You just might discover a new favorite food.

single one of them has been designed to serve a certain purpose for you and your body. Here are a few tips when it comes to understanding the fruits and vegetables in your fridge:

- **Not all fruits, veggies, and bodies are created equal.** This means that even though a fruit or vegetable has certain health properties, it might not sit well with your specific body. In chapter 3, I give the breakdown of fruits and vegetables and how they correlate to your health and mood. Use that
- **Quality of food vs. quantity of food.** It's important to understand the role quality foods plays in your health. Choosing quality food over large quantities of food will keep you healthier and feeling fuller longer.

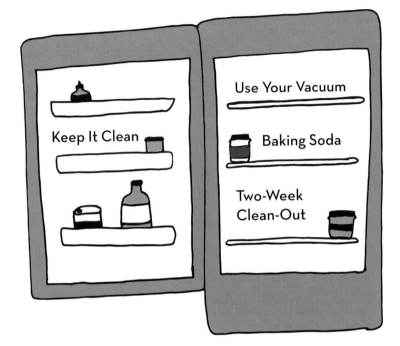

KEEP IT CLEAN

1. **Use Your Vacuum:** If your vacuum has a small attachment, use it to get crumbs and dried veggies at the bottom of your drawers. This is a great way to keep it clean and tidy!
2. **Baking Soda:** Keep an open box of baking soda in the fridge to help absorb any odors.
3. **Two-Week Clean-Out:** Clean out your fridge every two weeks—not just to keep it organized, but also to avoid having to throw out a ton of moldy produce every other month. But if you stop by the grocery store every few days, you may find yourself needing to throw out old produce and leftovers less and less often.

KEEP IT FRESH: A Quick Guide to Lasting Produce

SPOILED ROTTEN: PRODUCE THAT SPOILS FAST (1–3 DAYS)

Artichokes

Asparagus

Avocados (depending on how ripe they are when you get them!)

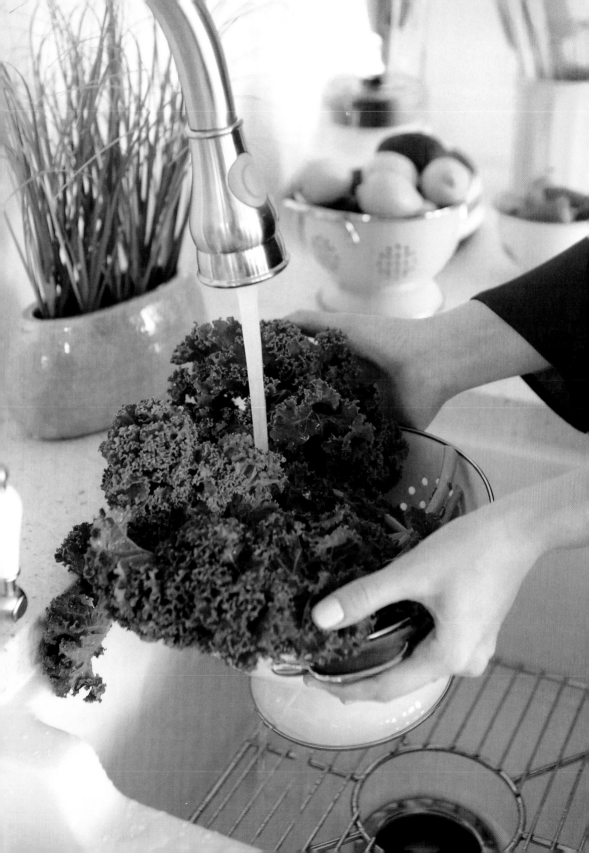

Berries
Broccoli
Corn
Mushrooms
Mustard greens
Okra

GIVE IT SOME TIME: PRODUCE THAT LASTS 3-5 DAYS

Arugula
Bananas—when you purchase yellow
    (If green, they will last a little longer.
    Too ripe? Make my PB Banana Chip
    Muffins recipe on page 160.)
Cantaloupe
Cucumbers
Eggplant
Grapes
Kohlrabi
Kumquats
Leafy greens, generally
Mangoes
Melons
Nectarines
Papayas
Peaches
Persimmons
Pineapples
Plantains
Radicchio
Zucchini

A WEEK'S WORTH: PRODUCE THAT WILL LAST ALL WEEK

Apricots
Bell peppers
Brussels sprouts
Cauliflower
Clementines
Grapefruit
Green onions
Heartier greens like kale and spinach
Kiwis
Leeks
Oranges
Pears
Peppers of other types
Plums
Tangerines
Tomatoes
Watermelon

WELL KEPT: PRODUCE THAT LASTS OVER A WEEK

Apples (6–8 weeks, if refrigerated)
Beets (2–3 weeks, if refrigerated)
Cabbage (3–6 weeks, if refrigerated)
Carrots (4–5 weeks, if refrigerated)
Celery (3–4 weeks, if refrigerated)
Cranberries (3–4 weeks, if refrigerated)
Garlic (3–6 months)
Onions, including shallots (1–2 months)
Parsnips (3–4 weeks, if refrigerated)
Pomegranates (several days at room

temperature and up to 3 months if refrigerated)

Potatoes, including sweet potatoes (2–3 weeks or until they spud!)

Radishes (7–10 days, if refrigerated)

Rutabaga (1–3 weeks, if refrigerated)

Squashes, whole (1–3 months)

Turnips (1–2 weeks, if refrigerated)

Meats and Proteins

MEAT AND SEAFOOD

When it comes to meat, the biggest factor in the equation is quality. It's better for your health, mood, and environment to eat high-quality meat less often than it is to eat low-quality meats more often.

Remember what I said about the energy of meat: If you eat a diet high in chicken, you may notice you become more anxious throughout the day, but cows tend to be calmer and more grounding, so you may crave beef if you had a crazy day and want to feel grounded again.

It's also important to recognize that you take on the energy of how an animal was treated. Choosing meats that came from loving environments and were fed a healthy diet will also help you digest, process, and feel good about the meat you are eating.

Here are a couple of tips when choosing meat and seafood:

- Choose organic local meats. When it comes to meat, local and organic is possible. Get to know your farmer or butcher and ask questions like:
  - What do you feed your animals?
  - How do you care for them?
  - Do your animals get hormones or antibiotics of any kind?
  - Do you name your animals? If so, what was this chicken's name? If you don't name them, can I call her Bertie? (Just kidding, don't ask that.)
- Avoid farm-raised seafood. Always choose fresh and wild-caught fish.

And if you can't get to a local farmer, butcher, or co-op, many conventional grocery stores (yes, even Walmart) are now selling meats from animals that were raised without added hormones, grass-fed, and sometimes organic. Opt for the best choice based on what your local market has available.

PLANT-BASED PROTEINS

A plant-based way of eating includes many protein options that can keep you healthy and sustained. Some examples include beans, legumes, quinoa, tempeh, and tofu. Here are tips when choosing plant-based proteins:

- Choose quality. Notice a theme? Always choose the highest-quality food possible. After all, your body deserves it.
- Make sure you're eating in balance. Most plant proteins don't contain all the essential amino acids to make a complete protein. When it comes to plant proteins, make sure you are balancing to get all the amino acids. For example, rice and beans together make a complete protein, which is why they're featured together in many vegetarian dishes. (Fun fact: Quinoa is the only plant-based protein that contains all the amino acids.)
- Avoid eating too much of one thing. Make sure you are eating a variety of foods. Sometimes plant-based junkies eat a whole lot of hummus, pizza, and tortilla chips and forget vegetables exist.

Food Mood Girl Love Note

Always listen to your body. Some people do well eating meat and others do not. We can all benefit from incorporating more plant-based meals into our diet.

Food Mood Girl Love Notes

Sprinkle a little black pepper on your eggs before serving to help balance the energy. You won't feel like you might crack. Pepper naturally helps awaken your digestive system almost immediately, making foods easier to digest.

- Be careful with soy. Too much of anything wreaks havoc on your health and your mood. Many plant-based products contain soy, and too much soy can disrupt your hormones and cause mood shifts. Make soy, like meat, a garnish and a treat rather than a staple.

EGGS

Nowadays you can get brown eggs, large eggs, extra-large eggs, cage-free eggs, organic eggs, non-GMO-fed eggs, free-range eggs, locally raised eggs, and eggs from chickens named Pamela. The reason there are so many types of eggs you can buy is because the regulations keep changing and the consumer demand to know where food comes from and how animals are raised is at an all-time high. The best eggs you can buy are from a local farm, where chickens have free

Fill a bowl with cold water and place the egg in the bowl. If it sinks to the bottom and lies flat, you have yourself a fresh egg. If it stands on one end, it's a little old, but still good to eat. If the egg floats to the surface of the water, then it is rotten and no longer edible.

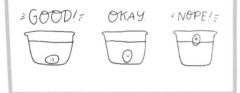

range and can do whatever the hell they want. Again, it all comes down to quality and care.

Just like meat, eggs carry a certain energy. Eggs can "crack" at any moment, and they are delicate, so a diet high in eggs might make you feel tense or on the verge of breaking.

Condiments

Ah, condiments. The things we buy, forget we have, and question if they are good or not the next time we go to use them. Condiments are a great way to flavor foods and add texture to dishes you

Avoid a Sticky Situation

When measuring out sticky foods like maple syrup, peanut butter, and honey, coat the measuring cups or spoons with a little olive oil or coconut oil. The ingredients will slip right out and leave you with virtually no mess!

create. Here is a quick guide to how long condiments last:

Ketchup: 6 months
Mustard: 1 year
Mayonnaise: The use-by date—usually 2–3 months
Hot sauce: 5 years (Thank God, because when I see my husband's two-year-old bottles, I cringe.)
Barbecue sauce: 3–4 months
Salad dressing: Use-by date or about 6 months
Salsa: If you buy the fresh kind, it can last 5–7 days. The jarred kind lasts about a month.
Maple syrup: 1 year
Honey: Never expires—seriously! It's the only food that doesn't!
Soy sauce or liquid aminos: 2 years
Jelly: 1 year
Olive oil: Best consumed within a year, but can last 2 years
Vinegar: 1 year

THE EASIEST SALAD DRESSING

Ran out of salad dressing? No problem! You can easily whip up your own healthy salad dressing at home. Use this simple ratio to create your new favorite go-to dressing:

3 parts oil + 1 part vinegar + your favorite spices

Check out the best oil to use for salads on page 103.

And remember, coconut oil does not make a great salad dressing because it hardens when it's cold. Instead, opt for olive oil and other low-heat oils to make your perfect dressing!

Dairy and Nondairy Alternatives

Cow's Milk: As with other meat products, ensure you are drinking the highest quality possible. Avoid milk with added growth hormones and antibiotics by checking the label. Many commercial milks will now say, "Does not contain growth hormones or antibiotics."

Cheese: Cheese is a food that tends to be all over the place as far as expiration. It really depends on the size, quality, and type of cheese. But for a rule of thumb, if it's moldy, then it's no good!

Also note that dairy does not work for everybody. If you are sensitive to dairy, try some of these alternatives instead.

Nut Milk: Nut milk—such as cashew milk, almond milk, Brazil nut milk, etc.—can be made by blending nuts and water and using a cheesecloth to drain. It lasts about 3–5 days in the fridge. See the nut milk recipes on page 151.

Coconut Milk: Coconut milk is another great dairy-free alternative that can be made with a can of coconut cream or shredded coconut. It can last 3–5 days in the fridge. See the recipe on page 151.

Leftovers: Store your leftovers in glass containers for up to 4 days. Keep them close to the front of the fridge so you eat them first!

The Staples

These are the must-haves for easy cooking and preparation anytime. With these simple ingredients, you will be able to easily whip up meals and snacks in no time.

DRY GOODS

Olive oil
Vinegars
Canned beans
Lentils
Chicken, beef, or vegetable stock and/or bouillon
Marinara or pasta sauce in a jar
Pesto in a jar
Coconut milk
Maple syrup
Honey
Grains such as rice, quinoa, and rolled oats
Canned tomatoes
Tomato paste
Pumpkin puree
Baking powder
Baking soda

REFRIGERATOR GOODS

Eggs
Milk (dairy or nondairy)
Butter (or nondairy butter)
Parmesan cheese

FROZEN GOODS

Frozen veggies (especially spinach, broccoli, and peas)
Frozen fruit (especially bananas and berries)

FRESH PRODUCE THAT "GOES A LONG WAY"

Potatoes
Carrots
Onions
Lemons
Garlic

THE MOOD ENHANCERS (SPICES)

Spice, spice, baby!

Spices are a chef's best friend. Not only can spices provide various minerals and mood-boosting benefits you need, but they can also create various flavor palates for your unique tastes.

Here is a list of common and mood-boosting spices to add to your pantry!

SPICE NAME	QUICK BENEFITS	HOW TO COOK WITH IT
SEA SALT	Helps balance the body's electrolytes, especially after exercise.	Use it to season your favorite dishes and enhance natural flavors.
BLACK PEPPER	Helps enhance your body's ability to obtain nutrients from food.	Add at the end of the cooking process as it loses flavor if cooked too long.
BASIL	Helps combat stress and improve heart health.	Use in salad dressings, bake in hearty dishes, or add to curries.
CARAWAY	Helps prevent bloating.	Best used in breads, soups, and sauces.
CHILI POWDER	Helps promote insulin regulation.	Spice up your favorite soups, stir-fries, and salad dressings.
CILANTRO	Helps reduce anxiety and fights against oxidative stress.	Best as a garnish or in fresh and raw dishes.
CINNAMON	Helps regulate blood pressure.	Helps bring out the natural sweetness in dishes. Best used in small amounts.
CORIANDER	Helps reduce inflammation and control blood sugar levels.	Toast lightly before adding to dishes like sautés or soups.
CUMIN	Helps the digestion process.	Add to soups, curries, and spicy dishes. Add to bean dishes to help reduce gas.
CURRY POWDER	Helps reduce pain and inflammation.	Add to your favorite curry dishes.
DILL	A natural energizer.	Dill pickles, duh! Great with fermented foods or added to fresh dishes.
FENNEL SEEDS	Can help combat bad breath.	Add to vegan dishes to bring out a sausage flavor.
LEMONGRASS	Can help alleviate stomachaches.	Best in marinades, stir-fries, and curry dishes.

SPICE NAME	QUICK BENEFITS	HOW TO COOK WITH IT
OREGANO	Can help boost the immune system and kill off bacteria.	Perfect to add to salad dressings or pasta/pizza sauces.
PARSLEY	Helps reduce inflammation.	Add to raw salads, sauces, and salad dressings.
ROSEMARY	Can help heal skin conditions.	Perfect with meats, potatoes, soups, or breads.
SAGE	Can help alleviate symptoms of depression.	Add to heartier foods such as meats, breads, and grain dishes.
SMOKED PAPRIKA	Can help improve your eye health.	A versatile spice that can be used to add flavor to vegetables, meats, grains, and beans.
SUMAC	High in omega-3 fatty acids, which can help improve your memory and brain health.	Best for salads and curry dishes.
THYME	Can help alleviate a sore throat.	Great for adding flavor but not overpowering a dish. Can be used in pasta sauces, breads, soups, and salads.
ZA'ATAR	This mixture contains mood-enhancing and brain-boosting properties.	A Middle Eastern mix that can be used in salads, meats, and vegetables.

SNACK ATTACK STATION

Every pantry needs a snack attack station. The last thing you want to do is "snackrifice" when you are standing in front of your pantry and asking a bag of stale popcorn to be a bag of tortilla chips and a side of guac. So keeping your pantry stocked with mood-boosting snacks that will satisfy every craving will help you to feel satisfied with your snack of choice and give your mood a boost as well.

This chart is a simple snack guide broken down by craving and mood. There is also space to list foods you enjoy in it.

Quit "snackrificing" and start living!

CRAVING	SAD	STRESSED	EXHAUSTED	HANGRY	BORED	FAVS
SWEET	Berries Orange Banana	Cantaloupe Carrots Figs	Apple Pineapple (grill it for extra flavor!) Mango	Pear Raisins Carrot sticks	Clementines Dates Pecans	
SALTY	Avocado toast Bean Salad Grilled mushrooms	Almonds Quinoa salad Sweet potato fries	Olives Grass-fed beef jerky Sunflower seeds	Scrambled eggs Herb-infused artichokes	Pickles Seaweed Roasted eggplant	
CREAMY	Green smoothie Oatmeal Salsa	Black bean dip (dip some carrots!) Peanut butter Coconut yogurt	Guacamole Dark chocolate Applesauce	Dippy egg Almond butter Chia seed pudding	Nut butter (add a little to the dates!) Hummus (dip some tortilla chips!)	
CRUNCHY	Walnuts Granola Peppers	Cashews Pistachios Rice crackers	Broccoli Kale chips Roasted Brussels sprouts	Radicchio Fried quinoa Celery	Roasted chickpeas Pumpkin seeds Tortilla chips	
DRINKS	Turmeric tea or lemonade Tomato juice	Chamomile tea Coconut water	Ginger tea Matcha tea	Carrot juice Lemon water	Cucumber water 100% pure apple juice	

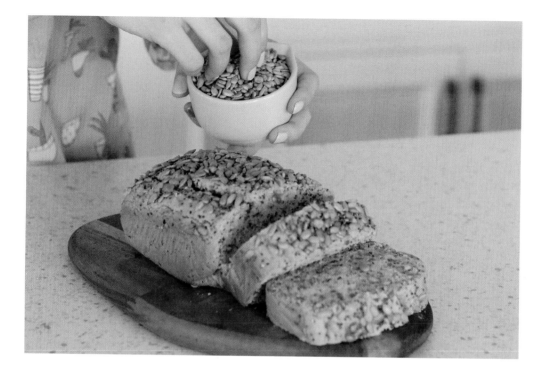

Snack Hack

Most people don't know that you can travel on a plane with food, just no liquids. Before you jet-set, ensure that you have some snacks on hand for those times when you might get hangry and the only thing in a fifty-mile radius is a vending machine. Also, if you are at a hotel, many times they have complimentary fresh fruit for their guests, so grab a few for the road if you find yourself pinched on time.

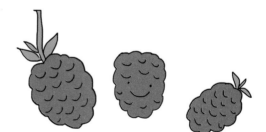

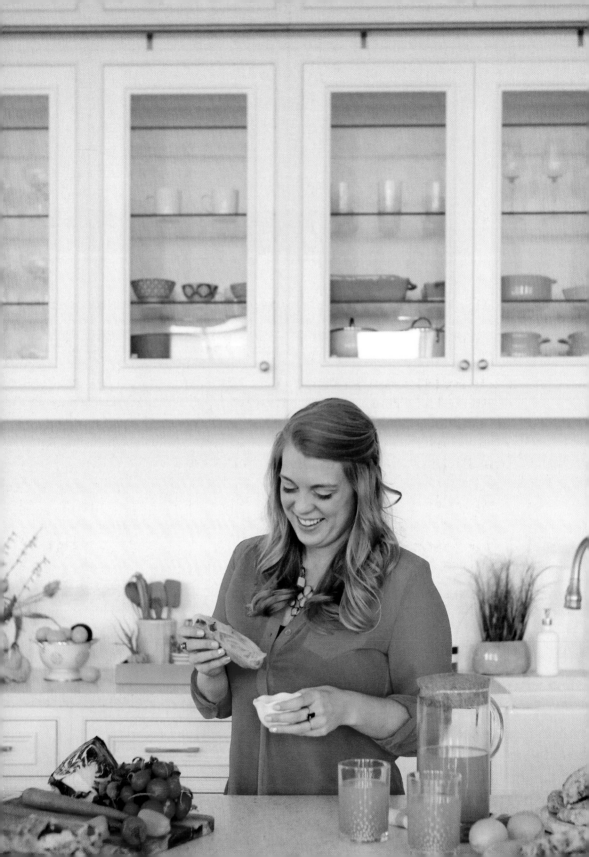

five

FOOD MOOD GIRL
COOKING BASICS

Now that we got all the technical stuff out of the way, we can start prepping to cook!

I got my first insight into the cooking world during my home economics class in middle school. Each week, we had to decide on a different recipe to make, depending on what skill we were learning. We then had to plan out how much of everything we would need, actually walk to the grocery store and get our items, and then finally prepare our dishes. I made everything from strawberry smoothies to casseroles to pumpkin pies. I fell in love with the art of cooking. I felt inspired knowing that I could take simple ingredients and spices and make something that tasted delicious.

I would often experiment at home, and throughout my high school years, I made my own lunches for school.

Then adulting happened. During college, I was working forty hours a week. Just the thought of having to cook something made me annoyed. I lost my cooking spark and eventually considered boiling water for noodles and heating up some sauce as cooking.

Before I switched careers to become a health and nutrition coach, I realized that the art of cooking was missing in my life. I had derailed so far from making my own lunches and truly feeling inspired by cooking.

So slowly but surely, I decided to reclaim my creativity in the kitchen. I started small, and each week I would try one or two new dishes. I started with recipes in cookbooks and eventually began experimenting myself.

Cooking is a creative expression, and once you allow yourself to be open to the possibilities and ideas that surround you, you will learn to love it.

I want to help you newbies in the kitchen get started. Remember, just one recipe a week can make a huge difference, not just for your health but also in your relationship with food and cooking. In the next few sections, I map out some of the basics of cooking. Once you learn and know how to prepare things (like how to properly cut an onion or how to use spices), you can take this knowledge to start creating dishes on your own.

You Are What You Chop!

I can think of many instances when the mere thought of chopping an onion or having to mince garlic made me want to just continue to lie on the couch, watch Netflix, and hope that food somehow miraculously appeared when I was hungry.

Most people enjoy cooking—they just don't enjoy chopping. It's not so much "you are what you eat" as it is "you are what you chop."

It seems basic, right? Know how to chop vegetables. But honestly, this is what holds most people back from attempting to cook in the first place, myself included.

Knowing HOW to use a knife and properly cut certain foods will empower you to get more involved in the kitchen and get excited to cook more often.

Knowing basic knife skills and how to cut the most cooking-friendly foods can help you feel like a major boss in the kitchen. If you know what to do going into it, you will feel more confident and are more likely to actually attempt a new recipe or even create one yourself. Below is an overview of your chef's knife and some basic handling and cuts you should know.

Let's get chopping!

How to Use a Chef's Knife

It's important to understand the various parts of the knife and how they work.

1. PROPERLY GRIP YOUR KNIFE

There are two steps to properly holding a knife:

First: Choke up on the blade with your thumb pressed into the top of the blade and your index finger on the opposite side. Wrap your remaining three fingers around the handle.

Second: Firmly hold your knife by gripping and wrapping your fingers around the handle.

2. POSITION YOUR GUIDE HAND

Positioning your guide hand is essential for kitchen safety. Make sure your fingers are tucked back and your knuckles rest against the side of the knife.

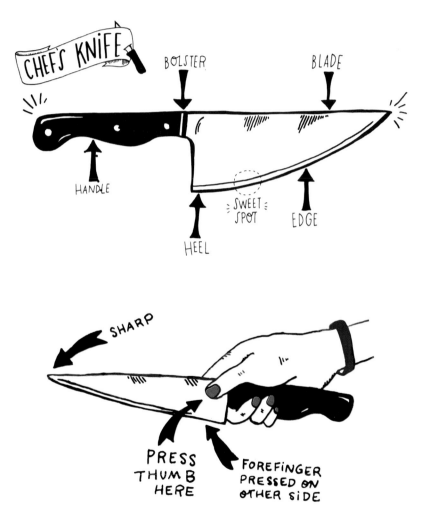

CHEF'S KNIFE

BOLSTER

BLADE

HANDLE

SWEET SPOT

EDGE

HEEL

SHARP

PRESS THUMB HERE

FOREFINGER PRESSED ON OTHER SIDE

3. GET COMFORTABLE WITH CUTTING TECHNIQUES

There are a few different cutting techniques you can use based on what you are cutting.

The Rolling Technique

This is the most popular of the cutting techniques. In this technique, the blade of the knife rolls through the food, with the point of the knife never leaving the cutting board. The tip of the knife is dragged back toward the food, the heel lifts, and then you push forward. Most of the cutting will happen on the sweet spot of the blade, or between the heel and the edge. Always make sure you have enough room on your cutting board to practice the rolling technique.

Variation: For larger cuts, you don't have to keep your knuckles against the blade, but you can instead place the knife farther down on the food since your cuts will be larger.

Up-and-Down Chopping Motion

For larger foods, you will have to take the knife off the cutting board in order to properly cut it. Use the center of the blade and anchor the knife against your guide knuckle. You will lose contact with your guide knuckle at every cut. You may also have to tilt the blade forward to ensure you can cut the entire food.

Pivot Chopping Technique

This is a variation of up-and-down chopping and is typically used for herbs. Anchor the tip in place with your fingers and rotate the knife as you chop. This will leave you with finely chopped herbs or other foods.

How to Properly Cut an Onion (and Avoid Runny Mascara)

If you are anything like I used to be in the kitchen, you cut an onion every which way, often ending up with half-assed and uneven onion cuts and tears rolling down your face.

But once you know how to properly cut an onion, your life will drastically change. You not only will know how to get the perfect cut you are looking for every time, but you also will know when you can cut for a good cry—or how you can avoid runny mascara altogether.

When you are trying to avoid runny mascara:

- Chill the onion in the refrigerator for fifteen minutes before you cut it.
- Light a candle while you cut. Not only does it set the mood, but the flame can help take some of the onion fumes away.

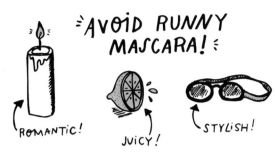

AVOID RUNNY MASCARA!

ROMANTIC!

JUICY!

STYLISH!

- Wear swimming or construction goggles. You'll look ridiculous, but your eyes won't burn.
- Rub lemon juice on your knife before cutting. This will help combat the onion juices from burning your eyes.
- Leave the root on when cutting. Most of the teary fumes are in the root, so keeping it intact will help prevent the burn.

And remember, if you need a good cry, do none of the above steps and let those tears out!

FOR SMALL DICES

1. Cut the pointy end off the onion and keep the root intact (unless, of course, you are in for a good cry; then take that off, too, and prepare for mascara to run).
2. Cut the onion in half through the root.
3. Peel the outer paper layer of the onion off.
4. Set one half of the onion on the flat side and make even cuts. Make sure not to cut through the root and instead use it to anchor the vegetable down.
5. Make perpendicular cuts to get nice and even dices.

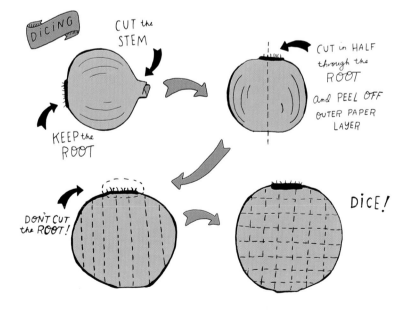

DICING

CUT the STEM

KEEP the ROOT

CUT in HALF through the ROOT and PEEL OFF OUTER PAPER LAYER

DON'T CUT the ROOT!

DICE!

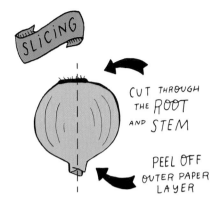

SLICING

CUT THROUGH
THE *ROOT*
AND *STEM*

PEEL OFF
OUTER PAPER
LAYER

LEAVE the
ROOT *intact*

FOR SLICING

1. Cut the onion directly down the middle, through the stem and the root.
2. Peel the outer paper layer of the onion off.
3. Start cutting slices at the stem, leaving the root end intact.

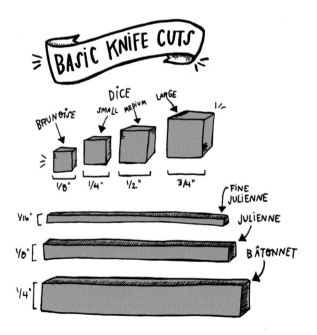

BASIC KNIFE CUTS

DICE

BRUNOISE   SMALL   MEDIUM   LARGE

1/8"   1/4"   1/2"   3/4"

1/16" [FINE JULIENNE

1/8" [JULIENNE

1/4" [BÂTONNET

EAT YOUR FEELINGS

DICE DICE BABY

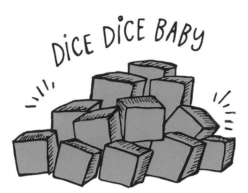

SMALL DICE: 1/4" x 1/4" x 1/4"
MEDIUM DICE: 1/2" x 1/2" x 1/2"
LARGE DICE: 3/4" x 3/4" x 3/4"

How to Cut a Pepper
THE JV WAY

1. Using a chef's knife, cut off the top of the pepper, just enough to remove the stem and expose the ribs of the pepper.
2. Hold the pepper and cut the ribs the entire way around the inside. Twist the ribs and pull out.
3. Cut the bottom of the pepper off and then cut the pepper in half lengthwise. You now have two rectangular pieces that you can julienne or dice.

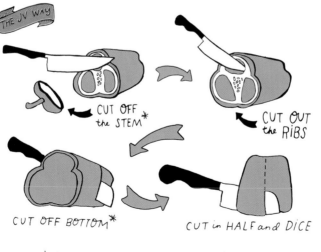

THE JV WAY

CUT OFF the STEM *

CUT OUT the RIBS

CUT OFF BOTTOM *

CUT in HALF and DICE

* DON'T FORGET to DICE THESE TOO!

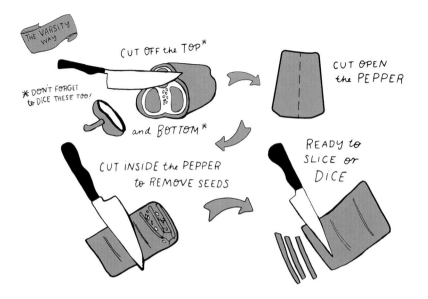

THE VARSITY WAY

CUT OFF the TOP*

* DON'T FORGET to DICE THESE TOO!

and BOTTOM*

CUT OPEN the PEPPER

CUT INSIDE the PEPPER to REMOVE SEEDS

READY to SLICE or DICE

THE VARSITY WAY

1. Using a chef's knife, cut off the top of the pepper, just enough to remove the stem and expose the ribs of the pepper.
2. Cut the bottom of the pepper as well, just enough to see inside the pepper.
3. Set the pepper on an end and use the tip of your knife to make one slice down to open up the pepper.
4. Now set the pepper on its side and use your knife to cut inside the pepper, with your knife blade parallel and facing away from you. Remove the ribs and seeds. Your pepper should now be lying flat.
5. Now you can cut the pepper into julienne slices or dice. Don't forget to use the top and bottom ends as well!

How to Mince Garlic

1. Place a garlic clove on a cutting board. Use the side of your knife and press down on the garlic clove. This will help naturally peel the paper off the clove and enhance the flavor.
2. Cut the garlic in thin strips from the root to the tip.
3. Turn the garlic 90 degrees and cut in the other direction.
4. Use the pivot chopping technique to go back and forth until it's as finely minced as you like.

Note: You can also opt for a garlic press!

Bonus Cuts (Because These Can Be Hard!)

HOW TO CUT AN AVOCADO

1. With your knife, slice the avocado lengthwise, around the seed, making sure to cut evenly on each side.
2. Twist the avocado until it comes apart in halves.
3. To remove the pit, there are two ways:

JV Option: You can scoop it out with a spoon, leaving as much avocado intact as possible.

Varsity Option: Gently tap the pit with the middle of your knife, just enough to slightly pierce it. Once the knife is secure in the pit, you can twist the knife to get the pit out.

HOW TO CUT A COCONUT

My favorite way to cut a coconut is . . . simply don't. But seriously, this one is a little tricky and may require actual tools such as a hammer. And by the time you get it done, you might end up hating coconuts. But if you are feeling ambitious or need to take your anger out on something, then by all means, attempt to cut a coconut! Grab your tool belt and get down to business.

1. First drain the liquid. Find the "eyes" of the coconut and use a corkscrew to puncture holes into the eyes. Drain the liquid.
2. Now, this is where you get to take out any aggression that you have. Place the coconut in a plastic or resealable bag. Place it on a concrete surface (a sidewalk will do!). From there, take a hammer and smash the coconut until it cracks.
3. Wonder why you just decided to do that.

HOW TO CUT A MANGO

1. Cut each side just past the seed so you get the flesh.
2. Slice the mango lengthwise without breaking the skin.
3. Use a spoon to scoop out the slices.

HOW TO CUT A PINEAPPLE

1. Place the pineapple on its side and cut through the top green crown.
2. Stand it upright and carefully cut the skin off from top to bottom.
3. You can now feel free to cut the pineapple as you wish!

Note: You can tell if a pineapple is ripe if it is easy to pull out a leaf from the top!

Kitchen Must-Haves

CULINARY TOOL	BENEFITS
CHEESECLOTH	You never know when you'll need one. Use this for straining homemade nut milks along with other culinary delights such as homemade ricotta and gnocchi. You can even use it to create a sachet for herbs to flavor home-made soups.
CHEF'S KNIFE	A proper chef's knife will help make almost any dish you need. Treat your chef's knife as your most prized tool in the kitchen and invest in one that you have tried and feel good about.
CUTTING BOARD	You are what you chop! So aside from a great chef's knife, it's also important to have a few cutting boards around. You want to make sure that your boards are big enough for what you are trying to cut. For example, you could use a small cutting board if you just need to cut a lemon, but you would need a large cutting board to cut an eggplant. P.S. Don't forget to oil your wood board with mineral oil to keep it clean and protected!
FOOD PROCESSOR	In a few seconds to minutes, you can process whole foods down to a meal or a liquid. Perfect for making nut flours and butters.
GARLIC PRESS	Makes it supereasy to mince garlic.
GLASS BOWLS	Use for mixing, adding to, and storing foods. Plastic bowls often contain BPA and other nasty additives that leach into food; glass does not.
HIGH-PERFORMANCE BLENDER, SUCH AS NUTRIBULLET OR VITAMIX	High-performance blenders excel at preparing soups, dips, smoothies, nut butters, and more. The NutriBullet is ideal for small batches and on-the-go smoothies. The Vitamix is great for family-size smoothies, batches of soups, and nut flours.
IMMERSION BLENDER	Easily mix and puree soups or mash potatoes right in the cooking pot. It eliminates the additional mess and cleanup of using a blender.
MANDOLINE	Whiz through slicing veggies like carrots, potatoes, and cucumbers. Makes veggie platters look unique so that crunching on veggies is fun.
RICE COOKER	The rice cooker changed my life. You can cook any type of grain, including oats. You simply put it on and prepare the rest of your meal while the rice cooks. It will let you know when it's ready, so no need to stare and check under the pot lid again.

EAT YOUR FEELINGS

CULINARY TOOL	BENEFITS
SALAD SPINNER	Wash and dry lettuce, spinach, or any other leafy green quickly and easily.
VEGETABLE SPIRALIZER	This gadget helps prepare vegetable pasta, such as zucchini or sweet potato pasta, easily and quickly. Check out the Zucchini Pasta recipe on page 246.

Types of Cooking

It's important to know the different kinds of standard cooking methods so that when recipes call for a specific type, you know exactly what is expected.

DRY-HEAT COOKING

Dry-heat cooking is when you apply heat either directly or indirectly to food. These methods include:

Broiling: Broiling is when you use heat from a source over the food, usually in the oven.

Grilling: Grilling is when you use heat from a source beneath the food. Think grills and charcoal.

Roasting: Roasting typically refers to cooking meats in a dry, closed heated-air environment, either in the oven or in an actual roaster. When roasting, temperatures typically start at 400 degrees or higher, giving food a browned outside.

Baking: Baking is when you surround food with dry heat in a closed environment. . . . It's best for fruits, veggies, meats, and baked goods. When baking, temperatures typically go no higher than 375 degrees.

Always Chop When Full

This is my personal motto because I can go from zero to hangry in the blink of an eye.

Sautéing: This is a transfer of heat using a small amount of fat, such as butter or oil. Best for cooking veggies and proteins.

Pan-frying: This is a mix between sautéing and deep-frying. Typically you use more fat than sautéing, and the food is often coated in a breading, batter, or flour.

Deep-frying: This is when you submerge the food into fat to cook.

MOIST-HEAT COOKING

Moist-heat cooking applies heat to the food by submerging it in liquid at various temperatures.

Poaching: This is when you place food in liquid, typically water between 160 and 180 degrees. The water should not boil, and there should be no bubbles. Keeping the temperature consistent is key. The most common item to poach is eggs.

Simmering: When you want to make food tender, you can simmer it by submerging it in liquid at about 185 to 205 degrees. This method of cooking can impact the food's flavor because you can simmer it in various broths or flavorings.

Boiling: This submerges food in hot and boiling liquid for a quicker cooking method. Boiling is most commonly used for vegetables and grains.

Steaming: This cooking method transfers the energy of steam to the food to cook it. Typically the food is placed in a steam basket above boiling water, which helps keep vegetables tender while maintaining the highest nutrient properties.

COMBINATION COOKING

Some cooking methods require a combination of both dry and moist heat.

Braising: This is typically used for large pieces of meat. You add enough liquid to cover the item halfway and heat it on the stovetop or in the oven.

Stewing: Stewed items typically are fully submerged in liquid, but are cooked at a lower temperature, around 300 degrees, until tender. Items are typically cut smaller and take less time to cook than braising.

Cooking Oils

There are a ton of oils out there, so it's important to know which ones are good for certain things. The last thing you want is to use coconut oil for a salad dressing, only to find it turns hard when you put it in the refrigerator and now becomes an Italian-flavored frozen-oil pop.

Here are the most common oils:

FAT/OIL	MOOD BENEFIT	APPROPRIATE HEAT PROPERTIES	HOW TO USE
EXTRA-VIRGIN OLIVE OIL	Helps keep your digestive track going and your hair and skin feeling nice!	Low heat	Use for salad dressings, low-heat cooking, or baking.
EXTRA-VIRGIN COCONUT OIL	Can kill yeast in your gut and give your brain and memory a boost.	Medium to high heat	Use for baking, sautéing veggies, stir-fries, pancakes, eggs, and more!
GRAPESEED OIL	Anti-inflammatory and helps reduce sugar cravings.	Medium to high heat	Use for baking, sautéing veggies, stir-fries, pancakes, eggs, and more!
SESAME OIL	Helps keep your skin clear.	Very low heat	Add last to stir-fries and other Asian dishes. Also use in salad dressings.
WALNUT OIL	Helps improve brain function and keep you from feeling fatigued.	Low to no heat	Drizzle onto dishes such as salads, vegetables, pizza, or even oatmeal.
FLAXSEED OIL	Helps combat symptoms of anxiety.	No heat	Drizzle onto dishes such as salads, vegetables, pizza, or even oatmeal.
AVOCADO OIL	Healthy fat and helps your body absorb nutrients in fruit and vegetable dishes.	Low to no heat	Drizzle onto dishes such as salads, vegetables, pizza, or even oatmeal.
BUTTER	Contains high levels of vitamin K2, which can help support heart and bone health.	Any heat	Great in baking and sautéing.

SOME THINGS TO NOTE ABOUT COOKING OILS

1. Buy oils in dark glass bottles. Clear plastic bottles are often mixed with various oils and can leach chemicals from the plastic into the oil.
2. Store away from the heat and light to help maintain its freshness.
3. Avoid vegetable oil and canola oil as often as possible as they are heavily refined and don't contain mood-boosting properties.

Moths Love Grains!

To help avoid a moth infestation, store your grains in the freezer. This will help kill any insects that might be in your grains and keep those pesky moths away.

Cooking with Grains

Whole grains are a pantry staple to make healthy dishes quickly and easily. Below are some of the most nutrient-dense grains available, complete with water-to-grain ratios and cooking times!

GRAIN	CUPS OF WATER FOR 1 CUP OF GRAIN	COOKING TIME
BARLEY	2–3 cups	1 hour
BLACK RICE	1.5–2 cups	1 hour
BROWN RICE	2 cups	45–60 minutes
BUCKWHEAT	2 cups	25–30 minutes
COUSCOUS	1 cup	5 minutes
FARRO	3 cups	30 minutes
FONIO	2 cups	3 minutes
POLENTA	3 cups	20 minutes
QUINOA	2 cups	15 minutes
ROLLED OATS	2 cups	20 minutes

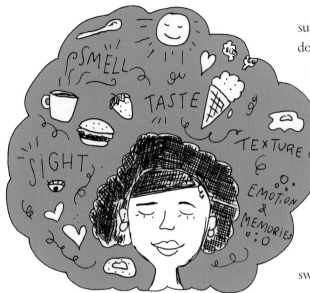

Food Mood Flavor Combining

AWAKENING YOUR SENSES

When you eat food, there are five main "senses" that are awakened.

1. Sight: You eat with your eyes first. How many times have you ordered something at a restaurant because you saw someone else eating it and it looked good? Everything about the presentation and packaging of a dish can affect whether we want to eat it.

2. Smell: The aroma of food can lure us into choosing a dish or a restaurant all by itself. Your sense of smell might be heightened as you walk past a bakery and suddenly you find yourself hungry for a doughnut.

3. Taste: There are five basic tastes when it comes to cooking and eating, and these are typically the flavors we are going over. These include sweetness, sourness, bitterness, saltiness, and umami (a Japanese word describing a savory, meaty, or "protein-y" taste). Oftentimes, these tastes show up in cravings such as "I want something sweet right now."

4. Texture: If you've ever had a conversation with someone about food, you've most likely heard him or her say, "I just don't like the texture." Texture can make or break a dish for us. Some people prefer foods like soup to be creamy and pureed, while others might like them a little chunkier and heartier.

5. Emotions and Memories: A trip down memory lane can trigger deeper emotions and awaken the senses. Suddenly your desire for a specific food or type of cooking is heightened and you find yourself wanting a specific dish to evoke that memory.

Keeping those key senses in mind can help you create dishes that hit all the components you want to achieve.

CULINARY FLAVOR COMBINING

Sometimes, we smell a spice or know we like it and add it to a dish only to find out the flavors don't actually go together.

This chart will help you navigate the best spices for the dishes you are trying to create based on various popular cultural culinary cuisines.

FLAVOR PROFILE	ITALIAN	MEXICAN	JAPANESE AND CHINESE	GREEK AND LEBANESE	THAI	INDIAN	AFRICAN
SPICES AND HERBS TO USE	Basil Chili Garlic Marjoram Onion Oregano Parsley Red pepper flakes Rosemary Sage Thyme Salt Pepper	Cilantro Cinnamon Chili Coriander Cumin Garlic Onion Paprika Parsley Saffron	Basil Cardamom Chili Coriander Garlic Ginger Miso Scallion Wasabi	Cilantro Cinnamon Chili Clove Dill Garlic Marjoram Mint Oregano Parsley Sesame Sumac Thyme Za'atar	Basil Chili Cilantro Coriander Cumin Curry Ginger Lemongrass Mint Tamarind Turmeric Sesame	Black pepper Cardamom Chili Cinnamon Clove Cumin Curry Masala Garlic Ginger Fenugreek Mint Mustard Onion Saffron Sesame Tamarind Turmeric	Cardamom Clove Chive Cilantro Cinnamon Coriander Cumin Garlic Ginger Mint Onion Saffron Sage
BEST FRUITS AND VEGGIES TO COOK WITH	Avocado Bell peppers Broccoli Capers Cucumber Olives Spinach Kale Lemons Tomatoes	Avocado Corn Chili peppers Jicama Limes Bell peppers Tomatoes Zuchhini	Broccoli Bell peppers Bok choy Cucumber Carrots Lemons Bean sprouts Seaweed Mushrooms Snow peas	Arugula Cucumber Eggplant Lemons Olives Pomegranate seeds Spinach Tomatoes	Carrots Cauliflower Coconut Peas Pumpkin Potatoes Tomatoes Zucchini	Bell peppers Cauliflower Coconut Eggplant Lemons Spinach Tomatoes	Bell peppers Cauliflower Corn Eggplant Lemons Melons Oranges Potatoes Tomatoes

FLAVOR PROFILE	ITALIAN	MEXICAN	JAPANESE AND CHINESE	GREEK AND LEBANESE	THAI	INDIAN	AFRICAN
BEST BEANS, LEGUMES, AND GRAINS	Arborio rice Barley Cannellini beans Fava beans Chickpeas	Black beans Brown rice Lentils Pinto beans Chili beans	Adzuki beans Barley Rice, including black, brown, and basmati Black beans Red beans Edamame	Chickpeas Lentils Barley Rice Quinoa White beans	Rice, including black, brown, jasmine, and basmati	Basmati rice Chickpeas Lentils	Basmati rice Fonio Chickpeas Lentils Millet Split peas
BEST OILS TO USE	Olive oil	Olive oil	Sesame oil	Olive oil	Olive or coconut oil	Olive oil	Olive or coconut oil
SAMPLE DISHES	Spinach Lasagna Soup (135) Sage, Sweet Potato, and Asparagus Risotto (137) Quinoa Pizza (145) Pistachio Chocolate Bananas (163) Easy Creamy Spinach (199) Pizza Scones (245)	Three-Bean Chili (138) Crusty Corn Bread (139) Nacho "Cheese" (142) Tasty Taco Salad (148) Guacamole (171) Chocolate Chia Seed Pudding (219)	Easy Hand Rolls (147) Asian Stir-Fry (168) Matcha Ice Cream (129)	Made-with-Love Brussels (197) Kohlrabi Slaw (205) Date Night Bites (219) Pumpkin Pie Hummus (226) Greek Salad (231) Cucumber Cups (229) Falafel Burgers (243) Za'atar Fries (243) Za'atar Salmon Bites (253)	Ginger Chip Cookies (132) Coconut Milk (151) Comforting Coconut Curry (164) Spring Rolls + Bowls (177) Mini Carrot Cake Muffins (239) Pineapple Peanut Noodles (247)	Spicy Butternut Squash Soup (173) Iced Turmeric Lemonade (183) Turmeric Tonic (183) Turmeric Milk Ice Cream (127)	Orange Cranberry Splash (152) Go-To Quinoa Salad (206) Simple Bean Salad (208) Cinnamon Pear Salad (225) Sweet Potato Fries (223) Roasted Cauliflower Mash (227) Power Wrap (230)

And if you don't feel like cooking . . . Order What You REALLY Want

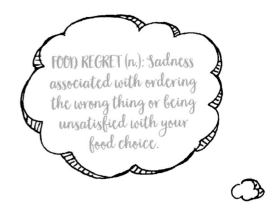

Oftentimes, when we go out to eat, or even in our home kitchen, we order and eat something because we think it's healthy and better than the thing we are actually craving. For example, if we go to a pizza joint, we'll order a salad because we think it's healthier and better for us. Meanwhile, all we really wanted was a slice of pizza. But we order the salad, eat it, and end up feeling unsatisfied. We really just wanted a damn slice of pizza.

What normally happens is your body then attempts to solve that pizza craving and you end up eating and snacking on a bunch of other random foods. So instead of eating two slices of pizza, you eat a salad with ranch dressing, half a box of crackers, a few slices of cheese, some tortilla chips and salsa, and a handful of pretzels. At this point, you should have just eaten the damn pizza. Not only would you have been satisfied, but you wouldn't have felt a need to binge later because your craving would have been solved.

Next time you go out to eat, allow yourself to order what you crave or feel called to. As you eat, savor the food and really enjoy it. Notice the smell, the flavors, and the textures. Chew slowly and mindfully.

Then notice how you feel later on. Do you feel satisfied with your choice? Did you eat it all, or were there leftovers? Did you binge on things later?

Experiment and notice how your body reacts when you go with your gut instinct with food choices or when you talk yourself out of it.

It's important to recognize this pattern in your food choices to help you release food regret and instead eat what your body tells you to.

Intuitive Cooking

Have you ever wondered how Grandma could go in the kitchen with no recipe and in an hour whip up the best meals and treats you've ever had?

You'd ask, "But, Grandma, where's your recipe?" And she would say that she doesn't use recipes.

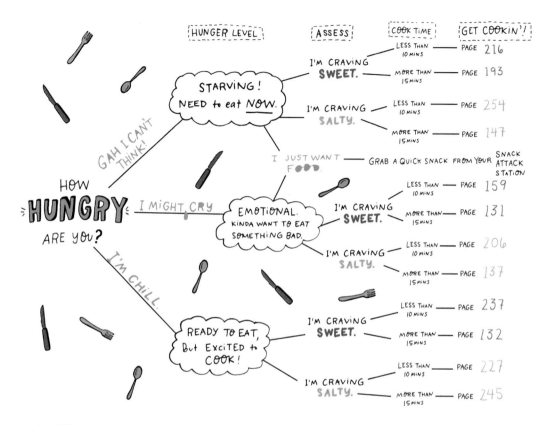

And if you are anything like me (recovering type A personality), this sends you into complete panic mode because you can't imagine cooking without a recipe. The mere thought of trying to create something without structure gives you more anxiety than you wish to have.

But Grandma knew something about food that we often forget. Food is truly a creative expression. From the way we cook and create recipes to the way we plate and showcase our dishes, it is all a creative act. It's a creative art form in which you use intuition, tasting, testing, and feeling to prepare something with love to share with others.

However, with perfectionist tendencies and the rise of convenience foods, we forget that cooking is an art form and often view it as a chore.

Choosing to see cooking as a creative adventure can help you shift your mind-set from "I can't cook anything" to "Let's get creative!"

To avoid inducing anxiety attacks, begin with a framework when cooking intuitively. That means starting with the recipe and following it to a tee. (Sigh of relief for all my fellow type A friends!) Follow every instruction and

FOOD + MOOD MAPPING

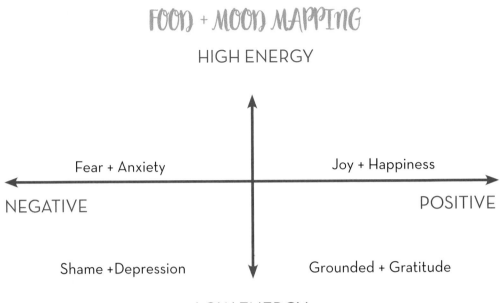

HIGH ENERGY

Fear + Anxiety   Joy + Happiness

NEGATIVE   POSITIVE

Shame +Depression   Grounded + Gratitude

LOW ENERGY

precisely measure every ingredient. A few days later, write down the recipe from memory and make it again. Do this a few times—except swap in ingredients that you like or spice combinations you want to change. Do this with several recipes and watch as you start to learn things about flavoring, combinations, texture, and what your palate enjoys.

As you start getting more comfortable in the kitchen, try incorporating one new vegetable a week. If something intrigues you, grab it and figure out what to cook with it. Start small by sautéing it or baking it. See what flavor comes out of it. You might find yourself saying, "Oh,

this would go really well in a sauté." Or, "Wow, I can really see this in a muffin." Start to trust your own gut instincts when it comes to cooking and flavoring.

The more you listen to your inner guide about food, the more empowered you will feel in the kitchen.

And the more empowered you feel in the kitchen, the better you feel and the better you eat.

Once you get more comfortable in the kitchen, use this food mood map of cooking to help you create your own dishes with no recipes needed.

It's also important to understand that all bodies are unique and amazing and that even fruits, vegetables, and healthy foods may not agree with some people.

I've developed the food mood mapping system so that you can create a unique plan that fits your body. It's important to complete a unique food mood map for your own body every six to twelve months as your body is constantly changing and evolving. Sometimes, what once made us feel great might not anymore.

It's about developing an intimate relationship with your body. After enough practice, you will know it so well that when you crave something or get sick, you can almost pinpoint the "what" and "why."

As you try different dishes or different foods, start to notice how you feel afterward. From there, you can start putting foods in categories based on your response to them. For example, what foods make you feel energized? What foods make you feel grounded? What foods make you feel anxious? Start adding foods to the mapping system so that you can better understand what your body needs to feel joy, happiness, serenity, or peace.

Food Mood Feeling Journal

Part of becoming a food-mood-etarian is discovering how you feel about what you eat. Each food can impact our mood in various ways just like our mood can dictate what we eat. Additionally, if you are stressed out and eat something healthy and still feel like crap, you might need to address the stress first rather than blame it on a kale salad.

It usually takes anywhere from one to three hours to feel the side effects of food, whereas if you are stressed, you might feel the side effects for hours on end.

Learning our bodies' intricate dance can help you discover how you can feel your best in mind and body. Some dances are easy to figure out, like the cha-cha slide or the Whip and Nae Nae, while others can be a little more challenging, like the tango. Be patient with yourself and allow your journey to be unique to you.

Use the journal below to help pinpoint what foods are working for you and which ones aren't. Journal for a week and check in with an audit. Notice patterns and get in tune with your foods and moods.

DATE	FOOD YOU ATE	HOW YOU FELT IMMEDIATELY AFTER	HOW YOU FELT AN HOUR LATER	HOW YOU FELT LATER IN THE DAY	OUTSIDE FACTORS (STRESS LEVEL, RELATION-SHIPS, ETC.)

WEEK ONE FOOD MOOD AUDIT

List of Foods I'm Jibing With:

_____

List of Foods I Should Let Go:

_____

Biggest Insight:

_____

One Reason Why My Body Is Amazing:

_____

EAT YOUR FEELINGS

Create Cooking Mantras

The energy we bring into our cooking experience gets infused into our dishes. It's no wonder food tastes better when you know it was cooked with love.

Practice cooking with fun mantras that you create and infuse each dish with a unique emotion. For example, if you want to feel more grounded, your cooking mantra could be "I am grounded."

If you want to feel like a Gloria Steinem, say "I am a badass feminist," and go cook with your badass self.

If you want to feel like Beyoncé, say "I am flawless."

The mantras can be fun, silly, funny, serious, or uplifting, whatever emotion you want to cook and eat with. Create your own to go with different dishes or change them up depending on your mood.

The One Ingredient They Don't Teach You About in Culinary School

There is a magical ingredient that can enhance the flavor of food without adding to the sugar, salt, or fat content.

This ingredient has the power to increase the nutritional value of the dish without compromising flavor.

This magical ingredient is love.

When you infuse love and happiness into your cooking, that ingredient carries through to your dishes, your plate, and the people who get to enjoy your food.

Figure out what energy you want to experience and cook with that energy. Do you want your meal to be a calming, energizing, or a peaceful experience? Visualize the end result and give each pour, scoop, stir, mix, and sauté the exact energy you want to get out of your experience.

You have the ability to add feelings of love, gratitude, and bliss into your food by transferring your energy to it. Dance while you are sautéing, sing while you are mixing, or simply listen to music and smile!

It doesn't matter whether you are preparing boxed mac 'n' cheese or crafting a homemade version; regardless of the food's nutritional value, cook with a positive and blissful energy. Not only will you have more fun in the kitchen, you'll also appreciate what you are eating, digest your food better, and even eat less because you get "full" on your energy.

Cook with your best attitude, and good energy will return to you.

Creating a Happy Home

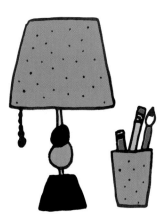 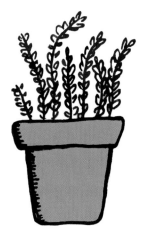

Since we spend a majority of our time in our homes, they should bring us joy and happiness rather than stress and anxiety. Changing your home environment can greatly impact your health and happiness.

When I walk into each room in my home, I think about how I want to feel. I then ask myself if the room makes me feel that way. Here are some of the questions I ask:

Does my office lift me up and inspire creativity?
Does my living room feel inviting to guests?
Does my kitchen get me excited to cook?

Does my air feel clean?
Does my bedroom feel comfortable and calming?
Does my bathroom feel clean, inviting, and relaxing?

If your answer is a "no" for any of those questions, it's time to focus on one room at a time to change the overall feeling and upgrade your area in order to achieve the joy you're looking for.

Here are some ways to spruce up your space to achieve certain desired moods.

How do you want to feel?

COMFORTED AND HAPPY

Best Colors to Infuse Your Space With
Pinks, browns, soft yellows

Tips to Spruce It Up

- Keep a nighttime gratitude journal on your nightstand. Every night before bed, write three to five things you are grateful for. This can help you sleep better and wake up feeling satisfied.
- Create a gallery wall of your favorite art and/or memories.
- Think simple. Oftentimes we want to fill our space with things so it doesn't look "bare," but simplicity is best.
- Clear your nightstand. Having a nightstand packed with random papers, books, and dusty candles will only make you feel more stressed.
- Add light to rooms. Oftentimes, we try to fill a room with furniture and extra art pieces, when in reality, it just needs some light, especially in dark winter months.

CALM AND CENTERED

Best Colors to Infuse Your Space With
Greens, blues, grays

Tips to Spruce It Up

- De-clutter your spaces. Anxiety can creep up when things are disheveled, so spend some time organizing the spaces that are most bothersome to you.
- Make your bed daily. If there is one space that should make you feel calm and centered, it's your bedroom. Plus, there is no better feeling than getting into a neatly made bed.
- Have a home technology zone. Reduce your screen time by having a designated room where technology happens (or doesn't happen!). That way, you can control the amount of screen time you get. Clear a space in your home for a little meditation spot with a comfy pillow or blanket that you can go to for peace, quiet, and reflection.

How do you want to feel?

ENERGIZED

Best Colors to Infuse Your Space With
Oranges, reds

Tips to Spruce It Up

- Adding live elements to your home can help make you feel more energized. Plants are a great way to feel alive and energized. If you are like me and tend to forget to water plants until they are wilting, then opt for some air plants or succulents, which require little care.
- Open your doors or windows when the weather is nice to allow a fresh breeze. Even in the winter months, I will make sure to crack my windows to allow some fresh energy into my space.
- Smudge areas of your home that need to be cleared with sage. Sage is a great cleanser of spaces and helps release any bad energy, allowing renewed energy to enter.
- Play music. Music is a natural mood booster. Extra bonus if you listen to music while cooking!

CREATIVE

Best Colors to Infuse Your Space With
Purples, oranges

Tips to Spruce It Up

- Add diffused essential oils such as lemon, grapefruit, and orange, which can all help lift creative energy.
- Create a vision board of your life's intentions. Add to it throughout the year.
- Add inspirational quotes to your desk or walls. Have them serve as mood-boosting reminders on days when you are feeling down.
- Create a creativity box. If kids can have a playroom, adults should at least have a creativity box. This box can include adult coloring books, paddleballs, yo-yos, stress balls, puzzles, card games, or any little fun items you can play with the next time you are feeling frazzled.

PURIFIED

Best Colors to Infuse Your Space With
Whites, blues

Tips to Spruce It Up

- Plants are a crucial life force that can help detoxify the air and cleanse your space. Adding low-maintenance and detoxifying plants to your house can help with your air quality and mood. Some of the best plants to keep around the house include:

  - Spider plant
  - Peace lily
  - Boston fern
  - Bamboo palm
  - Air plants
  - English ivy

- Essential oil diffusers can help purify your space and shift your mood depending on the scent.
- Air purifiers can make it easier to breathe.
- Home probiotics are typically sprays or machines that can naturally fight off bad bacteria and replaces it with good bacteria. This can help reduce allergies and increase your air quality.
- Water purifiers are a great way to purify your water and improve your health. You can opt for a whole-house system or use charcoal pitchers. Not only does the water taste crisp and clean, but you can be assured that the fewer chemicals you are getting, the better.
- Eco-friendly cleaning products can help reduce toxic exposure and make your house smell great. When switching out cleaners, I suggest starting with one and building your way up. Sometimes it might take trying a few different natural cleaners to see which ones you like best. You could also make your own using common household ingredients.
- Eco-friendly body care products are another way to purify not just your home but your body as well. As with the cleaning products, it's not necessary to throw out everything you own and replace with the new. Instead, start with one item at a time and work your way up. It might take some time to find certain products you love such as toothpaste, shampoo, and face cream. You can also try to make your own and see what you like best.

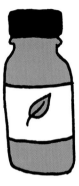

Craving-Kicker Roller

Small roller
Fractioned coconut oil
5–7 drops ylang-ylang essential oil
5–7 drops orange essential oil
5–7 drops bergamot essential oil
5–7 drops lemon essential oil

1. Fill the roller three-quarters of the way to the top with fractioned coconut oil.

2. Add the essential oils. Add additional oil, if needed, and place the roller tip on the top.

3. Close, shake, and roll away the cravings.

Calming Pillow Spray

3-ounce glass or plastic spray bottle
Distilled water
30 drops lavender essential oil
20 drops lemon essential oil

1. Fill the bottle three-quarters of the way with the distilled water.

2. Add the essential oils.

3. Shake before using.

Charcoal Teeth Whitener

Clear jar
4 tablespoons charcoal powder
2 teaspoons sea salt
5 drops peppermint essential oil
Clear jar

1. Combine all ingredients in a small jar with an airtight lid.

2. Dip your toothbrush in water and then dip in the mixture. Brush and rinse. Use a dark-colored washcloth to wipe up any drips on your vanity.

Coconut Oil Toothpaste or Teeth Whitener

Clear jar
1 tablespoon coconut oil
2 drops peppermint essential oil

1. In a small jar combine coconut oil and essential oil.

2. Place on your toothbrush and brush teeth thoroughly, or place the mixture in your mouth, swish for 10 minutes, and then spit into a garbage can.

3. Rinse your mouth with water and enjoy your new pearly whites.

Increasing Your Mood (Sans Food!)

While food plays a huge role in your emotional and physical well-being, it is not the only thing that feeds us.

Understanding your food–mood relationship has just as much if not more to do with the other things that feed you that you cannot possibly get in a quinoa casserole. These things include your career/life's work, relationships, spirituality, physical activity, finances, and creativity.

If you are in a toxic relationship that is constantly dragging you down, chances are your stress levels are high, your self-esteem is shot, and your body is in constant fight-or-flight mode. Until the toxicity from the relationship is either addressed and solved or released, your body will still feel the stress and side effects no matter how many cups of chamomile tea you drink a day.

It's important to recognize the areas in your life that are causing you sadness, stress, anxiety, or even boredom and instead of filling the void with food, healthy or not, figure out ways you can feed those areas.

Do a check-in with the various areas of your life. Notice what areas could use improvement, which ones are causing you stress, and which areas are going really well.

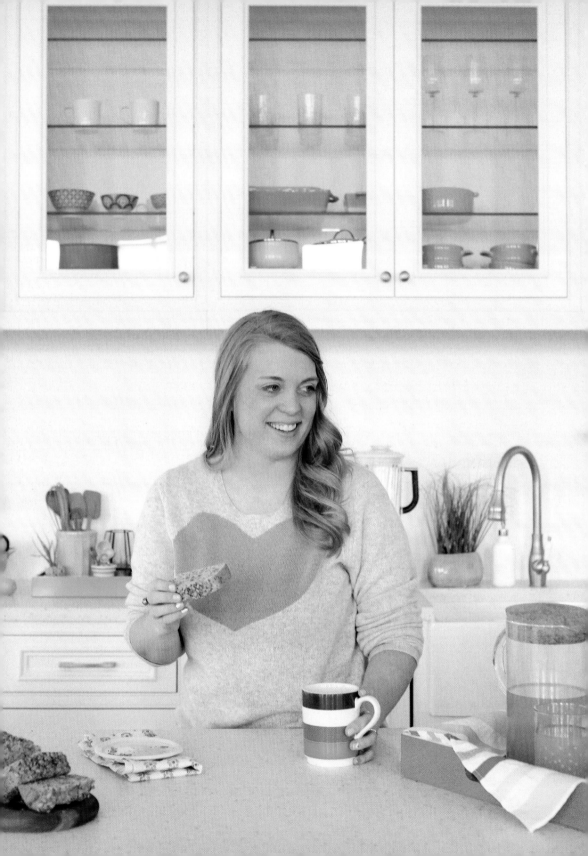

six

QUICK AND EASY RECIPES FOR EVERY EMOTION

Sad, stressed, or hangry? There is truly a food for every mood. Every food serves a purpose. And when I say "every food," I mean actual whole food, like fruits, vegetables, proteins, and whole grains. And while I, too, wish that those little gummy cheeseburgers and fries could be considered whole foods, unfortunately, they do not make the cut.

So anytime you are feeling sad, stressed, tired, hangry, or bored, simply go to this section and choose a recipe based on your craving.

While most of these recipes are plant-based, I also give optional additions where you can incorporate various meat proteins if you choose to do so. If you are gluten-free, you can substitute gluten-free flour, cup for cup, for any other flour. Like I said, there is a recipe for everyone, whether you eat meat or don't and whether you are gluten-free or not.

The goal of the recipes and lifestyle tips in these sections is to bring you to ultimate self-love and back to your happiest self.

And if you are feeling happy and hungry, any recipe will satisfy you and continue to increase your positive vibes.

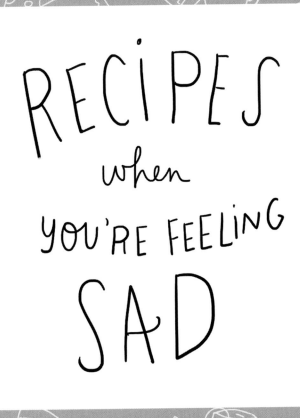

EMOTION: SAD

Regardless of our foods of choice, we sometimes reach to food to give us the sense of comfort or relief we are so desperately seeking. However, this usually takes us on a guilt-ridden roller-coaster ride. We feel sad, we eat junk—I personally reach for salt-and-vinegar chips—we feel guilt for eating junk, and then we are even sadder than when we got on the damn ride of despair!

While foods play a huge role in our emotions, it's important to understand that stuffing ourselves with either junk food or healthy food won't truly help us in the long run. It's important to first allow ourselves to feel our feelings of sadness. Experience the sadness or grief. It's not always fun, but it allows us to actually deal with the issues rather than reaching for food.

Once we embrace and accept our feelings, we can then start incorporating the right foods to help assist our every mood!

In this section, you will find which foods combat depression and sadness, accompanied by recipes for every craving that incorporate these happy foods.

It's perfectly acceptable to cry in this section—and not just when you are cutting those onions.

Create a Visual Dining Experience

The experience around eating can feed you just as much as the food itself. How does it feel to eat in a noisy subway station as compared to a quiet café? How does it feel to eat on a dining room table with papers and books piled around as opposed to beautiful place settings and candlelight?

The setup and surroundings you use to display and eat your food can light you up and make you feel happy before you even begin to eat.

Think about how you can create a creative, unique, and happy dining experience for yourself at home, on the road, and at work.

For Your Home: Try adding some colorful and eye-pleasing place settings at the table that make you feel relaxed and happy.

At Work: Try adding some fresh flowers to your dining area or eat outside when it's nice out.

On the Road: Try packing some fun utensils or place settings that are easily packable and accessible when traveling. When given a choice, try opting for an outdoor rest stop to enjoy your food or snacks.

SIGNS AND SYMPTOMS OF SAD EATING

- You have a "sad songs" playlist and listen to it on repeat.
- You are bummed out, and your first response is "I need to go get a candy bar."
- You find yourself crying while bingeing on ice cream.
- The thought of cooking brings you even more sadness.
- You skip food altogether because you feel too sad to cook.
- Doughnuts, pizza, and ice cream sound like a complete meal.
- There isn't any food! There are only ingredients to make food. The struggle is real.

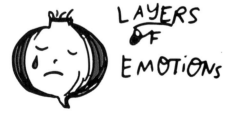

If you find yourself crying at a list of ingredients or sobbing over a direct email your boss sent, it's because your body wants to naturally release the stress and anxiety that accompany those hanger pangs. Crying helps stimulate the production of endorphins, which are feel-good hormones to help you go from sad to happy. So, while it sucks to cry at work or in a department store, it's really your body's way of saying "Don't worry, be happy."

WHAT'S (REALLY) HAPPENING TO YOUR BODY?

Whether you consciously know it or not, craving macaroni and cheese when you are sad has little to do with a physical craving or a lack of nutrients your body needs. It actually has everything to do with a memory.

Food evokes memories, both happy and sad. For example, I hated Indian food for the longest time because it reminded me of a blind date gone badly. Let's just say I forgot to mention I don't like superspicy things. Two bites into my rice dish, and I had snot running down my face like a toddler.

Aside from bad dates, food also provokes happy memories. Maybe anytime you were sick, your mom made you homemade chicken noodle soup.

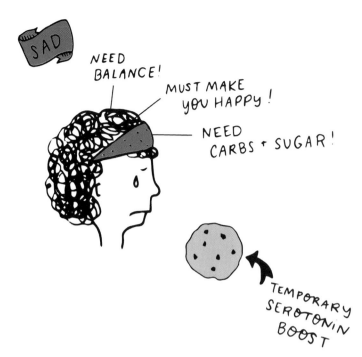

Or maybe every time you visited your grandma's house, she made peach pie for you. These memories shape the way we view foods. So if we are sad and need some comfort, we choose the things that gave us a certain feeling, one of happiness, comfort, calmness, or joy. It typically has little to do with nutrients or calories and more to do with memories and love.

There are, however, some physical things that are happening with your body. Aside from memories, your body is always attempting to find balance. If you are hungry, it wants you to feel satisfied. If you break a bone, your body wants to heal it. So when you are sad, your body wants you to be happy. Therefore, it hopes to find the pleasure-seeking chemicals found in food to help make you happy.

Typically people tend to gravitate toward carbohydrates and sugar because they can help increase your serotonin levels. However, they only increase it temporarily and then leave you to crash.

So when it comes to sadness and your food mood, it's important to first and foremost feel your feelings. If you are sad, don't immediately run to chocolate cake to attempt to fix your sadness, but instead acknowledge that it *is* okay to feel sad. Human beings are amazing in that way. We have a wide range of emotions we can feel on a daily basis, and sometimes feeling sad is okay and completely natural. So first acknowledge the sadness.

Then, once you allow yourself to feel the feelings, ask yourself what your body really needs. If you are craving something comforting like pizza or macaroni and cheese, then re-create one of the mood-boosting recipes in this chapter. Re-create those happy memories and fuel your body with ingredients that can physically help increase your happiness.

BEST FOODS KNOWN TO FIGHT OFF SADNESS

Asparagus
Avocado
Bananas
Beans
Berries
Cabbage
Celery
Grapefruit
Leafy greens
Mushrooms
Nectarines
Oats
Oranges
Quinoa
Raw cacao
Tomatoes
Turmeric
Walnuts
Watercress

Why These Foods?

Most of these foods contain special vitamins and minerals known to help prevent and alleviate the mood blues. Here are some of the key vitamins and minerals:

B Vitamins: B vitamins, specifically B5, B6, and B12 (especially combined with folic acid), can help regulate your mood and lift depression.

Omega-3 Fatty Acids: Fat is the new black. Days of the fat-free craze are behind us and we can finally embrace healthy fats. Healthy fats help boost your brain function by promoting new cell growth, which can help fight off sadness.

Tryptophan: Most people associate this chemical with turkey, but it's also found in a lot of plant-based foods. Tryptophan helps stimulate serotonin, which can help turn your rainy-day blues around.

Magnesium: This mineral helps develop serotonin, which is the feel-good neurotransmitter that can increase your happiness, along with your overall brain function.

OTHER TYPES OF FOODS TO EAT

Complex Carbohydrates: Foods such as whole grains, quinoa, rice, and sweet potatoes can help the body release serotonin, a feel-good neurotransmitter.

Gut-Friendly Foods: Since your mood and happiness directly rely on your gut health, gut-friendly foods such as fermented foods, low-sugar yogurts, and foods that contain probiotics can help you feel happier, too.

LIFESTYLE "FOODS"

It's also important to recognize the memory connection we have to food and how "feeding" your craving and increasing your happiness may have less to do with food and more to do with the memory. Try incorporating some of these lifestyle changes into your daily routine the next time you are feeling sad:

- Journal your feelings.
- Do an activity that fuels your memory. For example, if you are craving Grandma's apple pie, can you play a board game that you used to play with her instead or honor her memory in another way?
- Go for a walk. A simple ten-minute walk is enough to boost your mood and increase your happiness for up to two hours!
- Share your feelings with a close friend.
- Perform a random act of kindness for someone else. When you do something for someone else, it increases your empathy and helps you appreciate the good stuff in your own life.
- Take a shower or a bath. Sometimes cleansing yourself physically can help you feel better emotionally as well. Have a dance party in the shower or take a relaxing bath—whatever works for you.

WHAT TO DO WHEN YOU GET SAD

Wintertime SAD

Most people have heard of seasonal affective disorder, or SAD. When we hear this term, we immediately think of the wintertime blues. Usually, the cold temperatures and lack of sunshine can result in low vitamin D levels and a deflated mood.

In the wintertime, it's important to understand how you experience SAD and the types of things you can do about it. Here are some quick tips to help you relieve symptoms of wintertime SAD:

Vitamin D: Have you checked your vitamin D levels lately? Most Americans are deficient in vitamin D because it is nearly impossible to get adequate amounts of vitamin D from your diet alone. Sunlight exposure is the only reliable way to generate vitamin D. So in the winter months, when sunlight is low, our bodies have a harder time getting it. Vitamin D can help alleviate depression and naturally boost your mood, which makes it all the more important. During the winter months, it's extremely important to supplement vitamin D since your body has a harder time making it.

Light Box or Dawn Simulators: Light lamps and dawn simulators mimic outdoor light. Researchers believe this type of light causes a chemical change in the brain that lifts your mood and eases other symptoms of SAD. Using your box for fifteen to thirty minutes a day has been shown to "light" you up and get your day started on the right foot.

Movement: Make sure you get up and move throughout the day. If you don't feel like going to the studio or gym, try some simple exercises to get your body going.

Spruce Up Your Surroundings: Brighten up your home by adding lamps, giving the rooms some extra color, or enhancing your surroundings with some indoor plants. I am a huge fan of aloe vera and spider plants!

Summertime SAD

In the winter it seems as if most people are holding out for the summer. You may hear things like "I cannot wait for the beach!" or "I cannot wait for it to be nice out and not so gray."

While most people think SAD and wintertime go hand in hand, seasonal affective disorder can actually impact people in the summer, too. In fact, nearly a tenth of people who experience seasonal affective disorder feel their depressive symptoms in the summer.

The reasons why people experience summertime SAD vary, but some factors include body-image issues, the excessive heat, intense FOMO (fear of missing out) with all the activities going on, financial worries because of all the vacations, weddings, and events, and ever-changing, inconsistent schedules.

Here are a few things you can do to prevent summertime SAD:

Cool Your Engine: Think of your body as an engine. If you are someone with high energy or are prone to anxiety, your body is naturally hot, whereas if you are fairly calm and low-energy, your body is naturally cool. In the summertime, if you

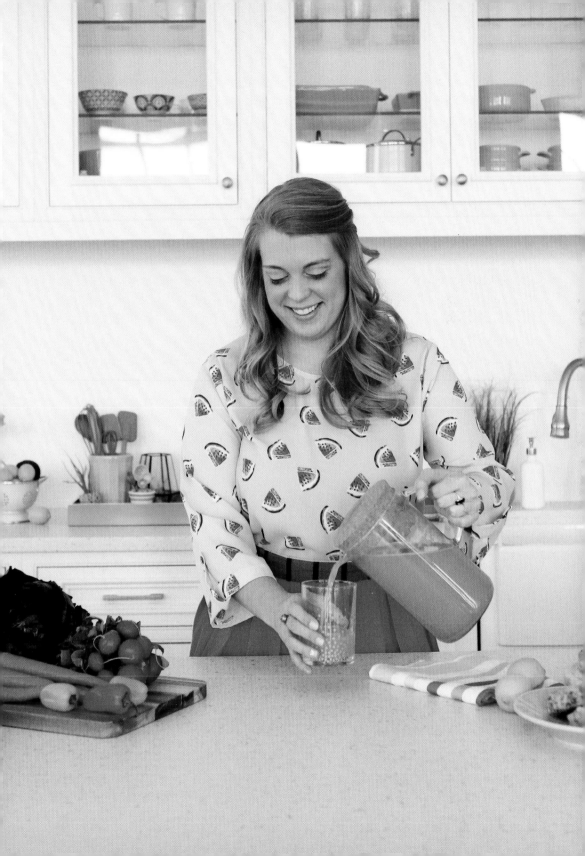

go to start your engine when it's already hot, it will overheat. The same is true for your body. So during the excessive heat in the summer, it's so important to cool your engine. If you work from home and don't have air-conditioning, try working at a coffee shop a few days a week. You may also want to take a dip in the local pool or even take a cooling shower. Not interested in doing any of that? Simply dip your feet in cool water for fifteen minutes to help your body naturally cool down.

Keep Hydrated: Well, duh! Right?! I know this sounds supersimple, but when you experience SAD in the summer, oftentimes you have zero appetite and this can include forgetting to drink water.

Have a filled water bottle with you at all times to ensure you are drinking throughout the day. This will help keep you cool and keep your brain functioning well.

Plan Your Life Accordingly: I know not everyone who experiences SAD can stop their entire life in the summer and wait until fall to be active again. However, knowing this, you can take proactive steps to make sure that you give yourself some extra space in the summer or finish any big projects before the heat has an impact on you. If you are planning a vacation, consider going somewhere a little cooler in the summer rather than hotter.

PB Chip Banana Ice Cream

Servings: 2
- 1 peeled and frozen banana, frozen in chunks
- ½ cup almond or coconut milk
- 1 tablespoon peanut butter
- 1 tablespoon dark chocolate chips or dairy-free chocolate chips

1. Blend the banana, milk, and peanut butter in a blender or food processor until smooth and creamy.

2. Depending on your level of sadness, you can choose to top with chocolate chips and eat immediately, or you can freeze for 30 minutes to give it more of a hard ice cream consistency.

3. Put your favorite funny movie on and enjoy!

Turmeric Milk Ice Cream

Servings: 2
- 1 peeled and frozen banana, frozen in chunks
- ½ cup coconut milk
- ½ tablespoon turmeric
- Dash of cinnamon
- Dash of black pepper

1. Blend all ingredients in a blender or food processor until smooth and creamy.

2. Eat immediately, or freeze for 15 minutes to give it more of a hard ice cream consistency.

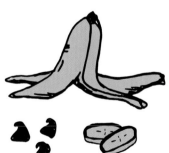

Breakup Ice Cream

In almost every breakup scene in modern-day movies, there's a woman sobbing into a pint of Ben & Jerry's.

I hate to break it to you, but when you are sad, your body is not necessarily ice cream deficient.

Instead, it's in need of some TLC and you typically won't find it at the bottom of a pint of ice cream. The ice cream is a temporary fix for an emotional hunger that, unfortunately, will never be fed with several scoops of brownie batter ice cream. And I know, I'm still dreaming of the day when we all wake up and this is true!

So before you hit the ice cream, try phoning a friend instead. Sometimes good company and a listening ear can treat you in ways that ice cream just can't.

If you are still craving something sweet, make your own breakup ice cream that will not only satisfy your ice cream craving but will also keep your mood stabilized, rather than leading to a crash the way store-bought ice cream can.

Matcha Ice Cream

Servings: 2
- 1 peeled and frozen banana, frozen in chunks
- ½ cup almond or coconut milk
- 2 teaspoons matcha powder

1. Blend all ingredients in a blender or food processor until smooth and creamy.

2. Eat immediately, or freeze for 15 minutes to give it more of a hard ice cream consistency.

NO ICE CREAM MAKER?
No problem! Fill a gallon-size resealable bag with ice and rock salt. Then take a sandwich-size resealable bag and add your ingredients to it. Place it in the large gallon-size bag and shake it like a Polaroid picture. After about 10 minutes, you will have creamy ice cream that you can eat right out of the bag.

BONUS TIP: If you don't want to make the ice cream with a banana, you can instead mix 1–2 cups of milk, the matcha powder, and 2 tablespoons maple syrup and use an ice cream machine to create your sweet and creamy treat.

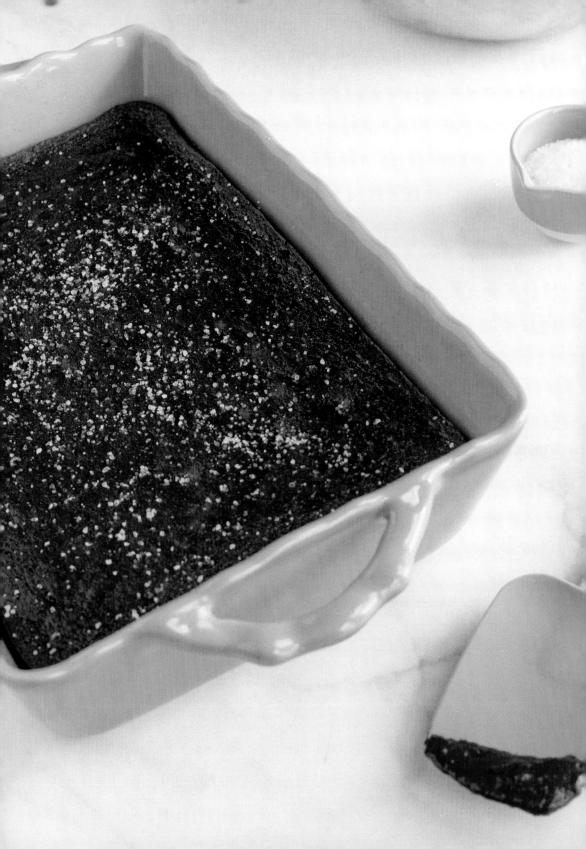

Dark Chocolate + Sea Salt Brownies

Brownies are the seventh wonder of the world. Well, kind of.

Servings: 12-16
  2 cups almond meal
  1½ cups raw cacao
  ½ teaspoon baking soda
  1½ cups maple syrup
  1 cup applesauce
  ½ cup coconut oil
  3 eggs
  2 teaspoons pure vanilla extract
  Sea salt

1. Preheat oven to 350 degrees.

2. In a large bowl combine your dry ingredients (excluding the sea salt) and mix. In a small bowl combine your liquid ingredients.

3. Slowly add your liquid ingredients to your dry mixture, and use a hand mixer to combine the ingredients. (If you are reading this and feel even sadder that you have to get a hand mixer out, it's okay, you don't really need one. A whisk, fork, or spoon will do. Just try not to get tears in the batter.)

4. Lightly grease a baking pan (an 11×7 or 8×8 pan works best) and add your batter, making sure it's even and smooth.

5. Bake for 25–30 minutes or until the center is fully cooked. Top with the sea salt and let cool. Enjoy with a tall glass of coconut or almond milk.

Note: If you want a lower-sugar brownie, use ½ cup maple syrup and 1½ cup coconut oil instead!

BONUS: These brownies taste delicious with the ice creams on pages 127 and 129!

Ginger Chip Cookies

Servings: 12 to 16

  2 cups almond flour
  ½ cup coconut palm sugar
  1 tablespoon ground ginger
  1 teaspoon cinnamon
  1 teaspoon baking soda
  Pinch of sea salt
  2 large eggs
  6 tablespoons melted butter or coconut oil
  1 teaspoon pure vanilla extract
  ½ cup dark chocolate chips

1. Preheat oven to 350 degrees.

2. In a large bowl combine your dry ingredients (excluding the chocolate chips) and mix. In a small bowl combine your liquid ingredients.

3. Slowly add your liquid ingredients to your dry mixture and use a hand mixer to combine the ingredients. Add in the chocolate chips and continue to mix.

4. Scoop about a tablespoon of cookie dough and place onto a lightly greased or parchment-lined cookie sheet.

5. Bake for 10–15 minutes or until the bottoms of the cookies are lightly browned.

6. Enjoy with a tall glass of coconut or almond milk.

Moody Bites

Servings: 12 to 15

  ½ cup coconut oil or butter
  ¾ cup maple syrup
  ¼ teaspoon sea salt
  2 teaspoons pure vanilla extract
  1 cup unsweetened dried and shredded
    coconut
  2 cups raw cacao powder

1. Blend the coconut oil, maple syrup, sea salt, and vanilla in a blender. If the coconut oil is solid, place it in a double boiler to warm gently first.

2. Add the shredded coconut ½ cup at a time and blend until smooth.

3. Transfer the liquid to a bowl and slowly add the raw cacao. Mix evenly until smooth.

4. Refrigerate 10–15 minutes to allow the mixture to set.

5. When the mixture has thickened, roll heaping tablespoons into balls.

6. Roll each ball in mood-boosting toppings (see below) and refrigerate until you're ready to serve!

INCREASE YOUR MOOD: Roll your Moody Bites in nuts, seeds, matcha powder, coconut shreds, or goji berries for an extra mood boost!

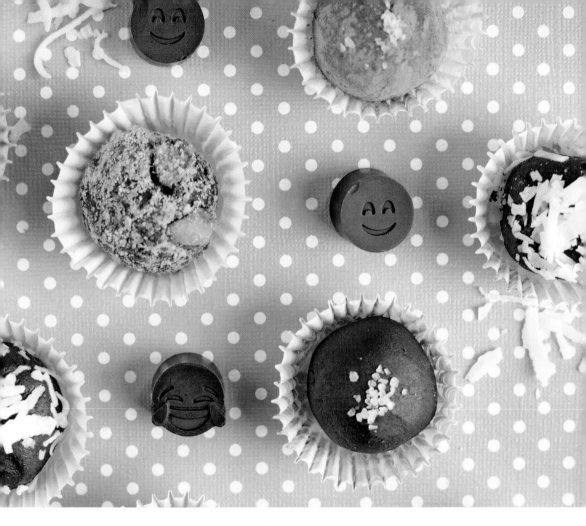

Emoji Chocolate

⅓ cup coconut oil
⅓ cup maple syrup
1 teaspoon pure vanilla extract
⅓ cup raw cacao

1. Blend the coconut oil, maple syrup, and vanilla in a blender. If the coconut oil is solid, place it in a double boiler to warm gently first.

2. Add the raw cacao and blend until smooth.

3. Slowly pour the mixture into a candy mold and freeze until solid.

4. Serve with the Moody Bites for extra mood-boosting pleasures.

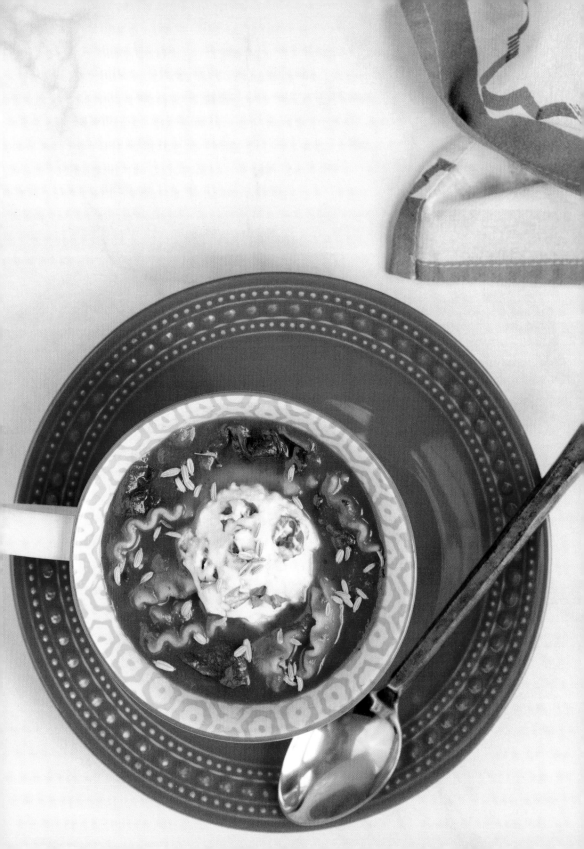

Spinach Lasagna Soup

Servings: 6 to 8

- 15 ounces ricotta cheese
- 1 cup shredded mozzarella
- 12 basil leaves, chopped
- 1 large onion, diced
- Olive oil
- 1 tablespoon fennel seeds
- 5 garlic cloves, minced
- 1 green pepper, diced
- 4 ounces fresh spinach (or 3 large handfuls)
- 28-ounce jar of marinara or tomato basil sauce
- 4 cups vegetable stock
- 1/8 teaspoon red pepper flakes
- 6 brown rice lasagna noodles
- Salt and pepper, to taste

1. For the topping, combine the ricotta, mozzarella, and basil in a small bowl and stir. Place in the refrigerator until the soup is ready!

2. For the soup, sauté the onion in olive oil in large saucepan on medium heat for 5 minutes.

3. Add the fennel seeds and garlic and continue to cook for another 5 minutes.

4. Add the green pepper and sauté for another 5 minutes.

5. Add the spinach and sauté until wilted.

6. Add the marinara sauce, vegetable stock, and red pepper flakes. Add the salt and pepper to taste. Bring the mixture to a boil and then let simmer for 30 minutes, stirring occasionally.

7. Break apart the brown rice lasagna noodles into 1-inch pieces and add to the soup. Cook for an additional 10–15 minutes or until the noodles are done.

8. Use a ladle to spoon the soup into a bowl, top with the basil and cheese topping, and eat up!

PROTEIN NOTE: Ground beef and sweet sausage taste best. Cook in a separate pan and add to the mixture 5–10 minutes before serving.

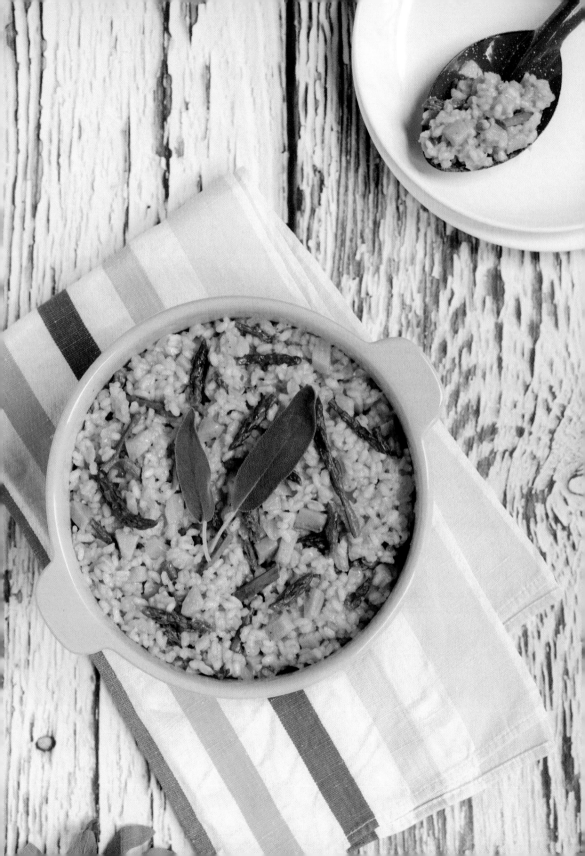

Sage, Sweet Potato, and Asparagus Risotto

Servings: 4 to 5

1 medium yellow onion, diced

4 garlic cloves, minced

1 cup Arborio rice

3 cups vegetable stock

6 sage leaves, chopped

2 small sweet potatoes, peeled and diced small

6-8 asparagus stalks, sliced

Olive oil

Salt and pepper, to taste

½ cup Parmesan cheese

¼ teaspoon red pepper flakes (optional)

⅓ cup pepitas

1. Preheat oven to 400 degrees.

2. On a baking sheet, lightly toss the sweet potatoes and asparagus with olive oil. Season with salt and pepper. Bake in the oven for about 25 minutes, tossing halfway through, cooking until both are golden brown.

3. In a large skillet, heat the olive oil over medium heat. Add the onion and toss for about 5–6 minutes, until it becomes translucent.

4. Add the garlic and cook for about 1 minute or until it becomes fragrant. Season with salt and pepper.

5. Add the rice to the pan and toss for a few minutes until the rice becomes translucent. Begin adding the stock ¼ cup at a time, and stir until the broth is absorbed. Keep stirring until the rice is al dente, about 25–30 minutes.

6. To finish the risotto, add the sage, sweet potato, asparagus, and Parmesan cheese and stir continuously. Add the red pepper flakes if you want a little heat.

7. Serve the risotto with the pepitas on top and indulge!

Three-Bean Chili

Servings: 4

1 large yellow onion, diced
Olive oil
6 garlic cloves, minced
1 large red pepper, diced
2 cans fire-roasted diced tomatoes
1 can black beans, drained and rinsed
1 can chickpeas, drained and rinsed
2 tablespoons chili powder
3 tablespoons cumin
2 tablespoons smoked paprika
¼ teaspoon red pepper flakes
1 cup vegetable stock
Salt and pepper, to taste

1. In a large saucepan on medium heat, sauté the onion in olive oil for 5 minutes.

2. Add the garlic and continue to cook for another 5 minutes.

3. Add the red pepper and sauté for another 5 minutes.

4. Add the fire-roasted tomatoes, black beans, chickpeas, chili powder, cumin, smoked paprika, red pepper flakes, and vegetable stock. Add salt and pepper to taste. Bring the mixture to a boil and then let simmer for 30 minutes, stirring occasionally.

5. Serve with a hunk of Crusty Corn Bread and enjoy!

PROTEIN NOTE: Ground beef and sweet sausage taste best. Cook in a separate pan and add to the mixture 5-10 minutes before serving.

Crusty Corn Bread

Servings: 6 to 8
  1 cup almond flour
  1 cup polenta
  ¼ cup chia seeds
  2 teaspoons baking powder
  ½ teaspoon sea salt
  ¼ cup coconut oil
  5 eggs
  2 tablespoons maple syrup
  ½ cup sweet corn, canned or fresh

1. Preheat oven to 350 degrees.

2. In a small bowl or food processor, combine the almond flour, polenta, chia seeds, baking powder, and salt.

3. Add the coconut oil, eggs, and maple syrup, and mix or blend until smooth.

4. Hand-mix the corn into the mixture.

5. Transfer the mixture into a parchment-lined or coconut-oil-greased cake pan.

6. Bake for 25–30 minutes or until the crust is golden brown.

7. Let cool and serve.

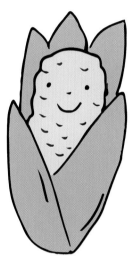

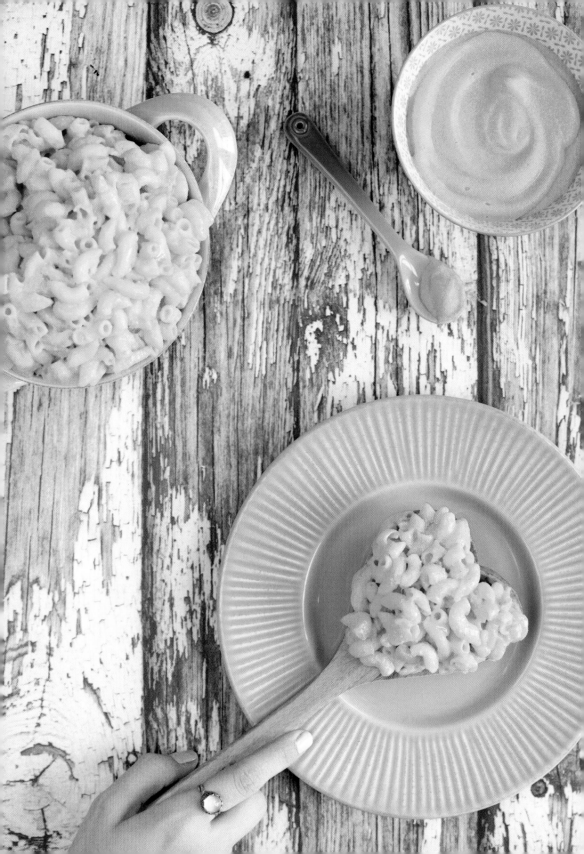

CREAMY

Mac and "Cheese"

Servings: 4 to 6

- 2 yellow potatoes, peeled and cut into 1-inch cubes
- 1 large carrot, cut into 1-inch chunks
- ½ white onion, chopped thick
- 1 bag of elbow pasta (I prefer quinoa or corn pasta!)
- ½ cup roasted cashews
- 1 tablespoon garlic powder
- 1 tablespoon onion powder
- 2 teaspoons sea salt
- 2 teaspoons black pepper

1. Bring a large saucepot filled with water to a boil and add the potatoes. Cook for 2–3 minutes.

2. Add the carrots and cook for 5–6 minutes.

3. Add the onion and boil for an additional 7–8 minutes or until the potatoes are soft.

4. While the vegetables are boiling, start another large saucepan and cook the pasta as directed.

5. Once the vegetables are done, remove them from the water with a slotted spoon and place in a high-powered blender. Make sure you save the water!

6. Add the cashews, garlic powder, onion powder, salt, pepper, and 1½ cups of the water into the blender. Blend until you get a smooth, creamy consistency.

7. Add the "cheesy" sauce to your elbow pasta, mix, and serve.

Nacho "Cheese"

2 yellow potatoes, peeled and cut into 1-inch cubes

1 large carrot, cut into 1-inch chunks

½ white onion, chopped thick

½ cup roasted cashews

1 tablespoon garlic powder

1 tablespoon onion powder

1 teaspoon cayenne pepper

2 teaspoons sea salt

2 teaspoons black pepper

1. Bring a large saucepot filled with water to a boil and add the potatoes. Cook for 2–3 minutes.

2. Add the carrots and cook for 5–6 minutes.

3. Add the onion and boil for an additional 7–8 minutes or until the potatoes are soft.

4. Once the vegetables are done, remove them from the water with a slotted spoon and place in a high-powered blender. Make sure you save the water!

6. Add the cashews, garlic powder, onion powder, cayenne pepper, salt, black pepper, and 1½ cups of the water into the blender. Blend until you get a smooth creamy consistency.

7. Dip in your favorite tortilla chip and you won't be able to tell you aren't really eating cheese.

Mushroom Melt Skillet

Servings: 2 to 4

1 tablespoon vegetable bouillon
   concentrate (or 1 cup vegetable stock)
½ cup quinoa
1 red onion, diced
Olive oil
4 garlic cloves, minced
8-10 Brussels sprouts, thinly sliced
1 cup oyster mushrooms, chopped
Salt and pepper, to taste
1 ounce chopped walnuts
1 ounce dried cranberries
½ cup Gruyère cheese, shredded

1. Preheat oven to 425 degrees.

2. Bring 1 cup water or the vegetable stock to a boil. If using water, add the vegetable bouillon concentrate. Add the quinoa, cover, and reduce to a low simmer for 15–20 minutes or until the quinoa is tender.

3. In a large cast-iron pan, add a drizzle of olive oil, add the onion, and toss until softened, about 4 minutes.

4. Add the garlic and toss for a minute or until fragrant.

5. Add the Brussels sprouts and toss until lightly browned, about 6–7 minutes.

6. Add the mushrooms and sauté an additional 5–6 minutes. Season with salt and pepper.

7. Once the quinoa is done, toss it into the cast-iron pan and mix. Add the walnuts and cranberries and mix thoroughly.

8. Sprinkle with the Gruyère cheese and bake for 5–7 minutes or until cheese is melted then serve!

PROTEIN NOTE: If you don't like mushrooms and want something meatier, substitute chicken for the mushrooms.

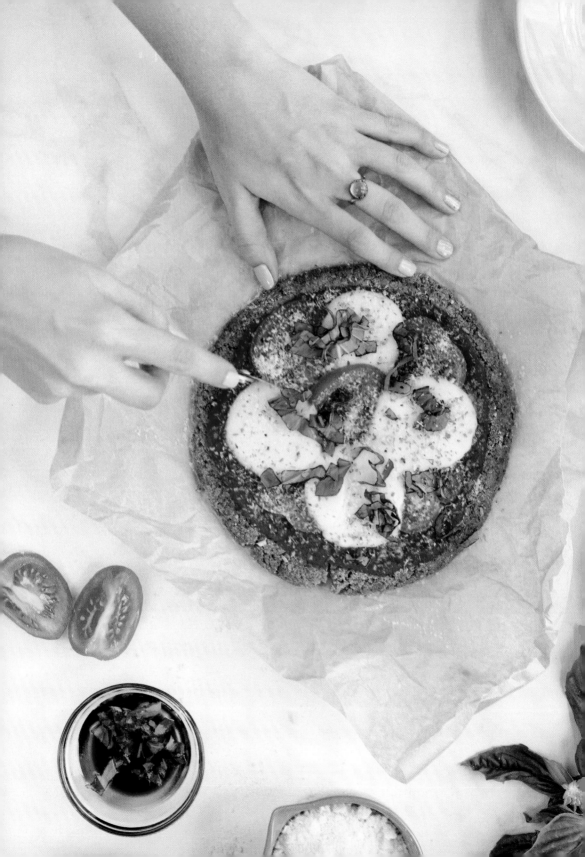

CRUNCHY

Quinoa Pizza

Servings: 6 slices

CRUST INGREDIENTS

1 cup quinoa (soaked for 5 hours)
1 tablespoon oregano
1 tablespoon garlic salt
½ tablespoon onion powder
1 tablespoon fennel seeds
Salt and pepper, to taste

OPTIONAL PIZZA TOPPINGS

Pesto + sun-dried tomatoes + buffalo
  mozzarella
Tomatoes + mozzarella + oregano
Fig jam + goat cheese + arugula

1. Preheat oven to 350 degrees.

2. In a food processor, combine the soaked quinoa, oregano, garlic salt, onion powder, fennel seeds, and a dash of salt and pepper. Blend until smooth and creamy.

3. Line a round cake pan with parchment paper and spread the mixture into the pan.

4. Bake for 12–14 minutes or until the bottom of the crust is light brown.

5. Remove and flip the crust onto a baking sheet. Top with your favorite pizza toppings.

6. Bake for an additional 10–15 minutes or until your cheese is golden brown.

Avocado Toast

Servings: 1

THE TRADITIONAL

1–2 pieces of sourdough bread
1 avocado
Salt and pepper, to taste

1. Toast your bread and spread with the avocado.

2. Sprinkle with salt and pepper and enjoy!

THE SWEETIE

1–2 pieces of sourdough bread
1 avocado
½ heirloom tomato, thinly sliced
1 tablespoon honey
Sprinkle of red pepper flakes

1. Toast your bread and spread with the avocado.

2. Add on the tomatoes, drizzle with the honey, and sprinkle on the red pepper flakes.

3. Wonder why you haven't had this type of avocado toast before!

THE SEEDY

1–2 pieces of sourdough bread
1 avocado
Sprinkle of hemp seeds
Sprinkle of chia seeds
Salt and pepper, to
   taste

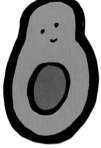

1. Toast your bread and spread with the avocado.

2. Sprinkle on the hemp seeds, chia seeds, and salt and pepper.

3. Enjoy every last bite!

Mini Egg Muffins

Servings: 18 to 24
  4 eggs
  ½ tablespoon sea salt
  ½ tablespoon ground black pepper
  ¼ cup diced onion
  ¼ cup diced bell pepper
  ¼ cup feta cheese
  6 basil leaves, chopped thin
  Coconut oil

1. Preheat oven to 350 degrees. Lightly coat the cups of a mini muffin pan with coconut oil.

2. In a medium bowl, beat the eggs. Stir in the salt and black pepper. Add the onion, bell pepper, feta, and basil.

3. Pour into the prepared muffin cups. Bake for 20–25 minutes or until the eggs are fully cooked.

Note: Swap in your favorite veggies, cheeses, and spices. Some of my favorites include:

  Sun-dried tomato, feta, and basil
  Cheddar and jalapeño
  Artichoke hearts and feta
  Potato and cheddar

Easy Hand Rolls

Servings: 4
  1 6-ounce can salmon (or tuna), drained
  ½ lemon, juiced
  Salt and pepper, to taste
  4 nori sheets
  ½ red pepper, sliced thin
  1 carrot, sliced thin
  1 avocado, sliced

EXTRAS

  Liquid amino acids, tamari sauce, or soy
    sauce
  Pickled ginger
  Wasabi

1. In a small bowl, break apart the canned salmon and season with salt, pepper, and the lemon juice.

2. Place your nori sheet on a flat surface and put a fourth of the salmon in a thin line down the middle. Add the red pepper, carrot, avocado, and pickled ginger and wasabi, if desired. Roll tightly.

3. Dip in liquid amino, if using, and enjoy!

FOOD MOOD GIRL LOVE NOTE: No nori? No problem. After you slice your avocado, keep the skins to use as bowls. Combine all the ingredients in a small bowl. Add ½ cup diced red onion. Place the mixture in the avocado skins and serve!

Tasty Taco Salad

Servings: 4 to 6

TACO "MEAT"

1 medium-sized white or yellow onion, sliced
8-10 shiitake mushrooms
1 cup walnuts
1 tablespoon cumin
1 tablespoon chili powder
1 tablespoon smoked paprika
½ tablespoon garlic powder
½ teaspoon salt
½ teaspoon pepper
½ tablespoon maple or coconut sugar
   (optional, if you like a little sweetness)
2-4 dashes cayenne pepper
Olive oil

RECOMMENDED SALAD COMBO

Spring greens
Tomatoes
Avocado
Salsa
Tortilla chips (for a little crunch on top!)

1. Start caramelizing the onion. Add about two tablespoons olive oil to a medium-large pan and add the onions, stirring to ensure all the slices are coated with olive oil. Cook on medium heat for about 30–40 minutes, continuing to stir every 5–10 minutes. The onion slices should caramelize and turn a nice golden-brown color.

2. While the onion slices are caramelizing, in a food processor, add the shiitake mushrooms and lightly pulse until they are shredded. Remove to a bowl and set aside.

3. Lightly coat a small pan with olive oil and toast the walnuts for about 4–5 minutes, turning as needed. Place them in the food processor and set aside.

4. Add all the spices to the walnuts in the food processor and process until finely ground. Mix into the mushrooms and set aside.

5. Once the onion slices are caramelized, stir them into the mushroom mixture. Lightly coat the same pan with olive oil and add the taco "meat" mixture, mixing in the pan for 4–5 minutes until crumbles form.

6. Create your salad! Start with the spring greens, add the taco mixture, top with the tomatoes, avocado, and salsa, and crunch a few tortilla chips on top.

Note: The taco "meat" in this recipe also makes great tacos. You can even make them into patties and fry for a burgerlike consistency.

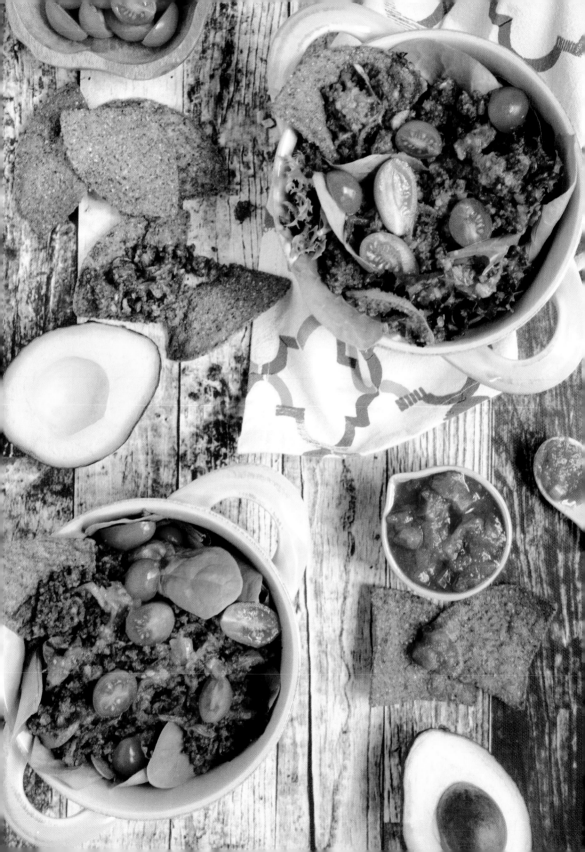

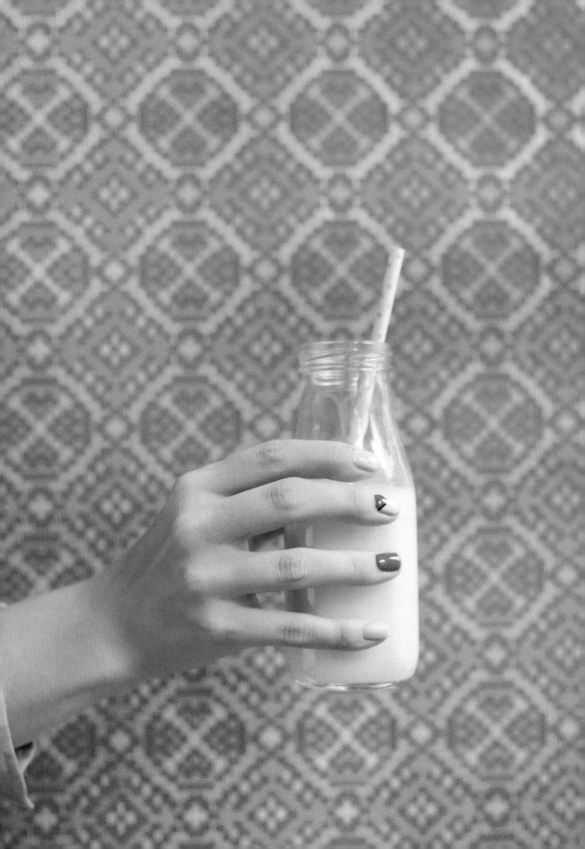

Nut Milks

Servings: 4 to 6

Coconut Milk

1 13.5-ounce can coconut milk
3 cups water
1 teaspoon pure vanilla extract

Blend the coconut milk, water, and vanilla on high for 10 seconds.

Hazelnut Milk

1 cup hazelnuts
3 cups water
1 teaspoon pure vanilla extract
Cheesecloth

1. Soak the hazelnuts for 3 hours, drain, and rinse.

2. Blend the hazelnuts, water, and vanilla in a high-powered blender until smooth.

3. Place a cheesecloth over an open jar and secure it with a rubber band.

4. Slowly pour the mixture through the cheesecloth and into the jar. If the cheesecloth gets full, remove and squeeze to get any excess milk into the jar.

5. Store for 3–4 days in your fridge!

Almond Milk

1 cup raw almonds
3 cups water
1 teaspoon pure vanilla extract
Cheesecloth

1. Soak the almonds for 3 hours, drain, and rinse.

2. Blend the almonds, water, and vanilla in a high-powered blender until smooth.

3. Place a cheesecloth over an open jar and secure it with a rubber band.

4. Slowly pour the mixture through the cheesecloth and into the jar. If the cheesecloth gets full, remove and squeeze to get any excess milk into the jar.

5. Store for 3–4 days in your fridge!

Note: If you like pulp or are feeling lazy, you can just blend and put into a jar. Shake before each use as the pulp will separate in the jar. This works well if you are using the milk for smoothies since it gets blended again then!

Moody Blues Smoothie

Servings: 1

1 cup raw kale
1 cup blueberries
1 ounce apple cider vinegar
1 tablespoon raw cacao
½ cup water or almond milk

Blend all the ingredients and enjoy!

Note: If you like your smoothies on the thinner side, try adding more liquid. If you like your smoothies thicker, reduce the liquid until you find the perfect blend for you.

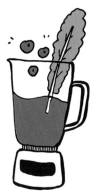

Orange Cranberry Splash

Servings: 1

1 tablespoon unsweetened cranberry
  concentrate
1 orange, juiced
16 ounces filtered water

1. In a large 20-ounce glass, combine the cranberry concentrate and orange juice and mix.

2. Add the filtered water, mix, and enjoy!

Tip: Just the scent of an orange is enough to give you an instant happiness boost. So this drink works twofold: first from the scent of the orange and second from ingesting the juice.

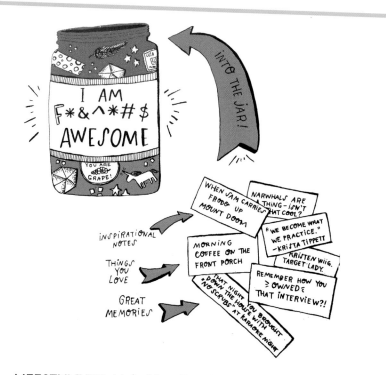

LIFESTYLE TIP: *Make Your Own "I Am F*&^*#$ Awesome" Jar!*

Instead of reaching for a jar of Nutella to demolish in one sitting, try grabbing an empty mason jar and making this "I Am F*&^*#$ Awesome" jar instead.

Simply decorate a mason jar with whatever makes you feel the best: feathers, mini unicorns, buttons, glitter, flowers, leaves, or cute dog photos you found on the Internet. Go crazy! The more fun you have with it, the better the chance of your mood lightening!

From there, write inspirational notes to yourself, your favorite funny quotes, nice things friends or colleagues have said about you, and even fun activities you enjoy doing. Fill the jar up as much as you can, and know that you can always add to it as inspiration strikes or whenever good things happen.

Keep this jar in your pantry, and the next time you are tempted to gobble down an entire jar of Nutella to drown your sorrows, try grabbing this jar instead! Sometimes a dose of self-love and a reminder of how f*&^*#$ awesome you are can help turn your frown upside down. No food needed.

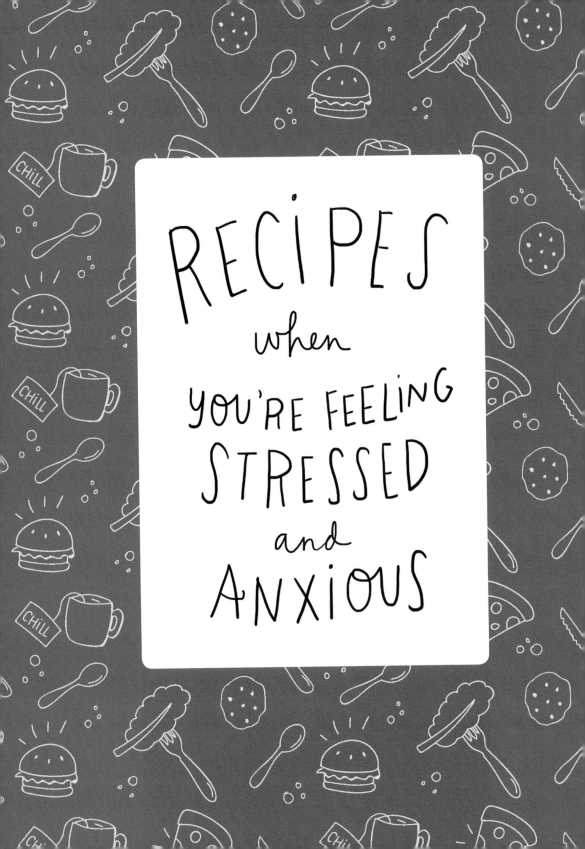

EMOTION: STRESSED AND ANXIOUS

Anxiety is the number-one mental illness in the United States, affecting about forty million Americans annually. Stress and anxiety can not only impact day-to-day wellness habits, such as sleep and energy, but it can also impact one's ability to leave the house, go out in public, or foster healthy relationships. Stress and anxiety both start internally but can then manifest physical symptoms. When you are feeling the daily stress and anxiety of life pile up, normally the last thing you want to do is grocery shop, prep food, and cook a meal.

As humans, we tend to want to choose pleasure over pain any day, which is why when we feel the stress of life, we tend to want to immediately do something that makes us feel good. And what better than a candy bar from the vending machine to give us an instant confidence boost?

We typically reach for foods that actually exacerbate stress symptoms rather than soothe them. For example, getting a midday cup of coffee might make us feel less stressed at the time, but it could lead to more anxiety and stress. Or reaching for something sugar-laden feels good in the moment, but only makes the crash and stress worse.

In this section, you will find recipes that can naturally help fight off stress and calm your body down so you can make decisions from a place of peace rather than chaos.

SIGNS AND SYMPTOMS OF STRESS EATING

- You pull off at the nearest gas station to grab a candy bar after work.
- It seems as if the vending machine is calling your name.
- You have an entire chocolate stash in your drawer and the only person who knows is you.
- You have an intense need to munch on something and don't know why.

STRESSED

GAH
I'M CRACKING
UNDER THE
PRESSURE!

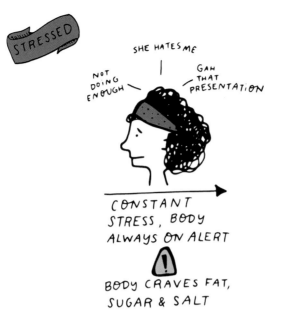

WHAT'S (REALLY) HAPPENING TO YOUR BODY?

When you are feeling stressed out, your body experiences the fight-or-flight response. So, for example, if someone was coming in to attack you, your body would trigger this response. Your blood rushes away from your stomach and into your head, hands, and feet because in a life-threatening situation, you need to be able to think quickly and either fight back or run away.

Chances are, you aren't getting into physical fights every day, but it is highly likely you are constantly fighting with your internal self. Everything from "I'm not doing enough" to "Is my boss mad at me, or is he/she going to like my presentation?" This type of stress is extremely toxic on the body because it induces low levels of stress over time. So rather than the one-off attack, where your body can go back to normal pretty quickly, this actually means that your body is on stress alert most of the time, never being able to return to normal.

When this happens, physically you may find yourself gaining weight, suffering from indigestion, and craving foods that you believe will bring you balance such as foods high in sugar, salt, and fat. In reality, these foods tend to only enhance your stress throughout the day.

While stress triggers are different for everyone, it's important to first address the biggest stresses in your life and see if there is something that can be resolved to help ease it up.

Life happens, and some days, stressful things are going to happen that are out of your control. However, if you can incorporate stress-reducing foods, healthy mind-set shifts, and techniques that help you calm your body, you will be able to handle any stressors that come your way.

BEST FOODS KNOWN TO FIGHT OFF STRESS

Almonds
Arugula
Asparagus
Avocados
Beets
Black beans
Cantaloupe
Carrots
Cashews
Chamomile
Coconut
Eggs
Figs
Fish
Leeks
Mushrooms
Oatmeal
Onions
Parsnips
Passion fruit
Peaches
Peanut butter
Peppers
Pistachios
Potatoes
Quinoa
Raspberries
Spinach
Squash
Sweet potatoes
Tempeh
Turmeric

Why These Foods?

Most of these foods contain vitamins and minerals that help combat your stress levels. Here are some of the vitamins and minerals to look for:

Magnesium: This vitamin is responsible for helping with everyday brain function, from tying your shoes to keeping your heartbeat steady without even thinking. Most people are extremely magnesium deficient, which can leave you feeling overwhelmed and stressed out.

GABA (Gamma-Aminobutyric Acid): This special neurotransmitter is responsible for shutting off brain activity. It's more or less responsible for helping you shut off your brain to fall asleep.

OTHER TYPES OF FOODS TO EAT

Grounding Foods: Foods that are grown in the ground can help you physically feel more grounded.

LIFESTYLE "FOODS"

You can drink as much chamomile tea and eat as many sweet potatoes as you want, but if you are constantly under stress, you need to do more than scarf down a bowl of sweet potatoes. Here are some lifestyle "foods" to incorporate:

- Go for a ten-minute walk to clear your mind.
- Grab an adult coloring book and color your favorite picture.
- Start a gratitude journal and write down three to five things you are grateful for every day.
- Practice the art of saying no. If something doesn't feel like a "HELL YEAH," then simply pass.
- Read a book for pleasure.
- Put on a simple meditation CD and take five minutes to meditate by yourself.

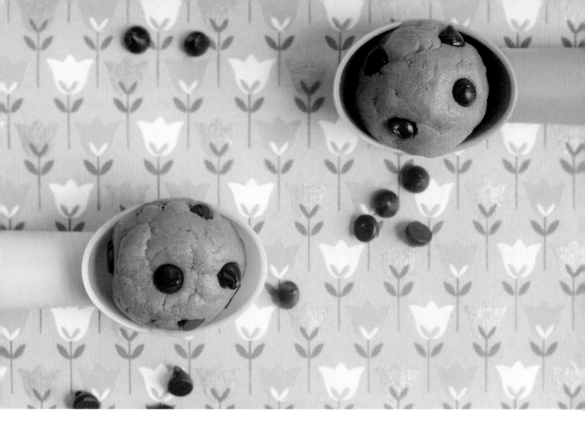

SWEET

Cookie Dough Contraband

Servings: 12 to 16
- ½ cup almond butter
- ⅓ cup honey or maple syrup
- 1 cup almond or cashew flour
- ¼ cup chocolate chips

1. Combine the almond butter and honey or maple syrup.

2. Add the nut flour and mix until a ball of dough forms.

3. Add the chocolate chips.

4. Roll into bite-size balls and freeze for 30 minutes.

Raspberry Bites

Servings: 6
  6 raspberries
  6 dark chocolate chips

1. Wash raspberries and dry.

2. Place a chocolate chip in the opening of each raspberry.

3. Enjoy this simple sweet treat.

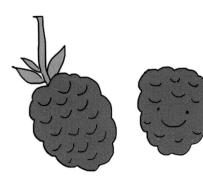

PB Banana Chip Muffins

Servings: 12 to 14
  2 large ripe bananas
  ⅓ cup coconut oil
  ⅓ cup maple syrup
  ⅓ cup peanut butter
  1 teaspoon pure vanilla extract
  1 egg
  1¼ cups nut flour, gluten-free flour, or whole
    grain flour, sifted
  Pinch of sea salt
  Chocolate chips, to your liking (I actually like
    fewer chocolate chips—weird, I know!)

1. Preheat oven to 350 degrees.

2. In a large food processor or blender, combine the bananas, coconut oil, maple syrup, peanut butter, pure vanilla extract, and egg. Blend until smooth.

3. In a large bowl combine the flour and salt with the liquid mixture until mixed thoroughly.

4. Fold in the chocolate chips.

5. Pour the mixture into lined muffin tins.

6. Bake for 12 to 15 minutes, until the

EAT YOUR FEELINGS

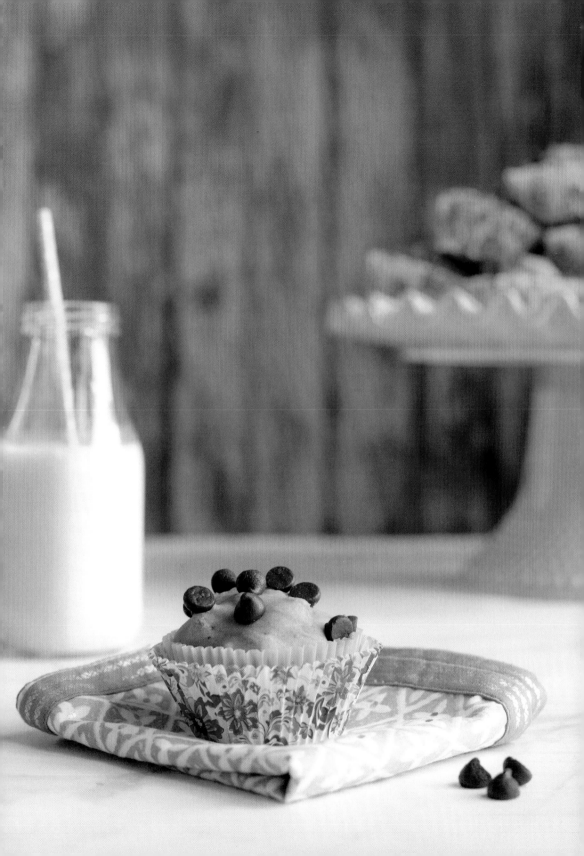

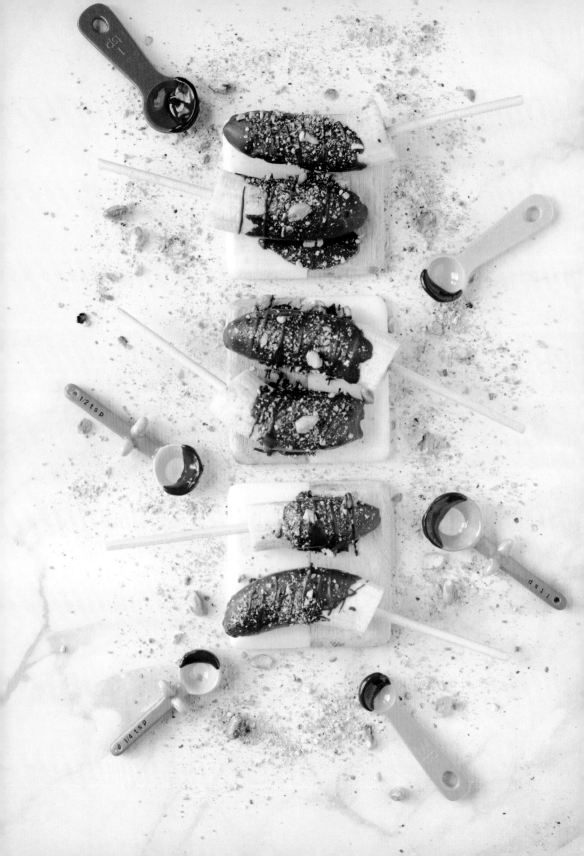

Pistachio Chocolate Bananas

Servings: 6

3 bananas
6 popsicle or cake pop sticks
Coconut oil
½ cup dark chocolate chips
½ cup pistachios, crushed

1. Line a baking sheet with parchment paper.

2. Peel the bananas and cut in half crosswise.

3. Insert a stick halfway into each banana half. Place in the freezer.

4. Add a little coconut oil to a small saucepan, put on low to medium heat, and add in the dark chocolate chips. Stir until melted, but make sure it doesn't burn.

5. Take the bananas out of the freezer, dip in the chocolate, and sprinkle the pistachios on top.

6. Freeze for at least 30 minutes more before serving.

BONUS: No chocolate chips? No problem! Use the Emoji Chocolate recipe on page 133 in place of melting chocolate chips!

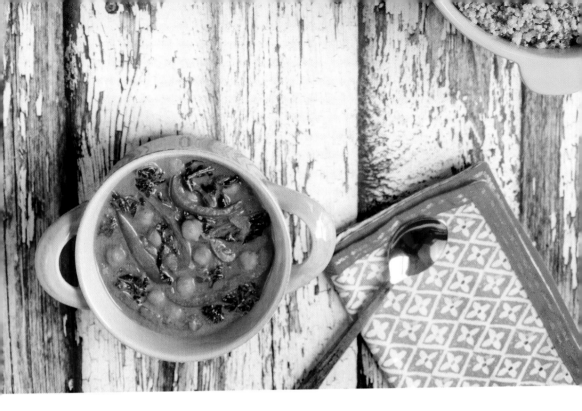

SALTY

Comforting Coconut Curry

Servings: 6

Olive oil

1 red onion, minced

Salt and pepper, to taste

6 garlic cloves, minced

1 bunch kale (approximately 6–8 stalks),
thinly sliced

4 tablespoons curry powder

1 teaspoon turmeric

1 tablespoon smoked paprika

1 13.5-ounce can coconut milk

1 cup vegetable stock

1 15-ounce can chickpeas, rinsed and
washed

1 red pepper, thinly sliced

5 Medjool dates, minced

1. Lightly oil a sauté pan and add the onion. Add a little salt and pepper and cook down until it is caramelized/browned.

2. Add the garlic and mix for about 30 seconds or until fragrant.

3. Add the kale and cook until it's wilted.

4. Add the curry, turmeric, and paprika and mix until the kale and onion are covered.

5. Add the coconut milk and vegetable stock. Allow to simmer on low heat for 10 minutes.

6. Add the chickpeas and red pepper and simmer for another 10–15 minutes.

7. Add the Medjool dates and stir. Simmer for another 10 minutes.

8. Serve over rice, quinoa, or your favorite grain!

PROTEIN NOTE: Add sautéed tofu 5 minutes before serving.

Slow It Down

How often are you running around all day, scarfing down food to get on to the next thing? When is the last time you actually stopped to chew your food or even thought about it?

Chewing is actually the first step in the digestion process, and it's crucial that you chew your food up in order to maximize your nutrients, give your digestive system a break, and genuinely feel fuller and satisfied.

Take a week to really practice the art of chewing. Try chewing your food until it is liquid. Notice how you slow down, how your body digests, and how satisfied you feel.

The act of slowing down and chewing not only aids in our digestion but also can help calm our nerves and give our bodies an extra boost of nourishment.

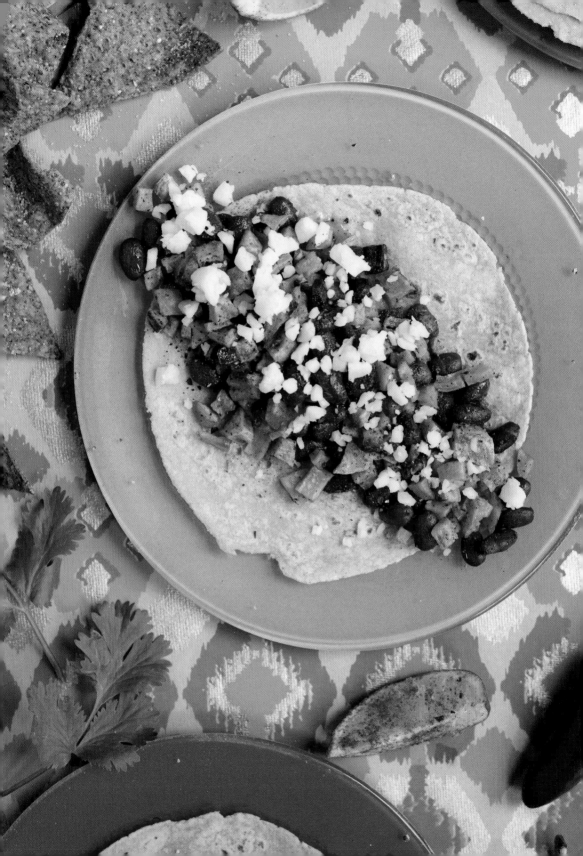

Sweet Potato and Black Bean Tacos

Servings: 6

2 sweet potatoes, peeled and diced small
Olive oil
2 tablespoons honey
1 teaspoon cumin
1 teaspoon chili powder
½ teaspoon cinnamon
⅛ teaspoon red pepper flakes
1 15-ounce can black beans, drained and
    rinsed
6 tortilla shells

OPTIONAL TOPPINGS

Feta cheese
Salsa
Cilantro
Guacamole (page 171)
Salsamole (page 227)

1. Preheat oven to 350 degrees.

2. Line a baking sheet with parchment paper and place the sweet potatoes on it. Lightly drizzle with olive oil and honey.

3. Combine the cumin, chili powder, cinnamon, and red pepper flakes in a small bowl, then sprinkle the mixture evenly on the sweet potatoes and toss.

4. Bake 10–15 minutes or until the sweet potatoes reach your desired texture. Halfway through the baking, mix them so you get even cooking on all sides.

5. In a medium skillet, heat the black beans for a few minutes, just enough to get them warm.

6. In a medium-size bowl, mix together the baked sweet potatoes and black beans, adding salt and pepper to taste.

7. Scoop the mixture onto the tortillas, top with your choice of toppings, and enjoy!

PROTEIN NOTE: Add a little cooked beef if you want a meatier taco. Avoid chicken as it can make you more anxious.

MAKE IT A TOSTADO!

If you are bored with tacos (although I don't know how you could ever be bored with tacos), make it a tostado instead. Simply take your tortilla and heat it directly over your stove flame. (Electric works, too.) Start with low heat and use tongs to continually flip it until it becomes hard and crunchy. Then layer your ingredients on the tostado and top with your favorite add-ons.

Asian Stir-Fry

1 cup quinoa, uncooked
Olive oil
1 yellow onion, diced
3 garlic cloves, minced
1 red pepper, sliced thinly
2 carrots, shredded
1 broccoli head, chopped small
¼ teaspoon red pepper flakes
2 cups spinach
4 tablespoons liquid amino acids (or soy sauce)
1 tablespoon sesame oil
Salt and pepper, to taste
4 eggs (optional)

FOR THE QUINOA

Use a rice cooker to get your quinoa started. Quinoa is a 2-to-1 ratio grain, so you need 2 cups of water for every cup of uncooked quinoa. If you don't have a rice cooker, bring a small pot with 2 cups of water to a boil. Add a little olive oil and 1 cup quinoa, reduce the heat, and cover for 15 minutes or until the quinoa is done.

FOR THE STIR-FRY

1. Lightly coat a large skillet with olive oil and heat over medium heat.

2. Add the onion and cook for 5 minutes or until translucent.

3. Add the garlic and cook for 2 minutes or until fragrant.

4. Add the pepper, carrots, and broccoli. Stir until all the ingredients are lightly coated, and cook for about 10 minutes.

5. Season with salt, pepper, and the red pepper flakes and stir.

6. Add the spinach and cook until wilted.

7. Increase the heat to medium-high and stir in the cooked quinoa.

8. Add your liquid amino acids and continue to stir.

9. Reduce the heat and drizzle the sesame oil over the stir-fry.

10. For an extra boost, serve with a fried egg on top.

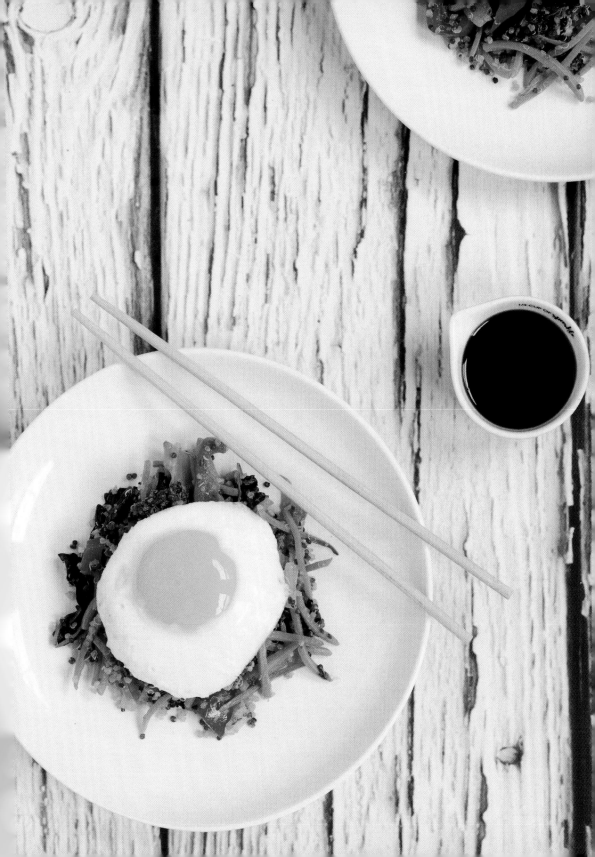

Sweet Potato Quesadilla

Servings: 2

1 small sweet potato
2 tablespoons coconut oil or olive oil
Pinch of sea salt
1 tablespoon ground cinnamon
¼ cup cooked black beans
¼ cup fresh pineapple, cubed
2 gluten-free soft-shell tortillas
¼ cup cheddar jack cheese

1. Preheat oven to 400 degrees.

2. Cut the sweet potato into chunks and place on a baking sheet. Lightly coat with the oil, salt, and cinnamon. Bake until tender, about 15 minutes. Once the sweet potatoes are done, increase the oven to 450 degrees.

3. Meanwhile, in a small skillet, combine the beans and pineapple. Heat for about 5 minutes.

4. Brush a little olive oil on one side of each tortilla and place one on a baking sheet. Top with the sweet potatoes, pineapple and bean mixture, and the cheese. Cover with the remaining tortilla, oil side up.

5. Bake for 6 to 8 minutes, flipping halfway through, ensuring the quesadilla is crisp and the cheese is melted.

PROTEIN NOTE: Add a little cooked beef or sautéed tofu if you want a meatier quesadilla. Avoid chicken as it can make you more anxious.

CREAMY

Guacamole

Servings: 3 to 4

3 ripe avocados
½ onion, diced
½ red pepper, diced
1 lime, juiced
Salt and pepper, to taste

1. In a medium bowl, mash the avocados with a fork.

2. Add the onion and red pepper.

3. Add the lime juice and salt and pepper to taste.

4. When I dip, you dip, we dip.

BONUS: Add pomegranate seeds for an additional mood boost.

Put the Pit in Your Guac!

To keep your guacamole nice and green all day before serving, save your avocado pits and add them to the dip to keep it from browning. Remove the pits before serving and no one will know what time you made it.

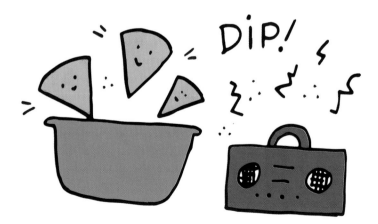

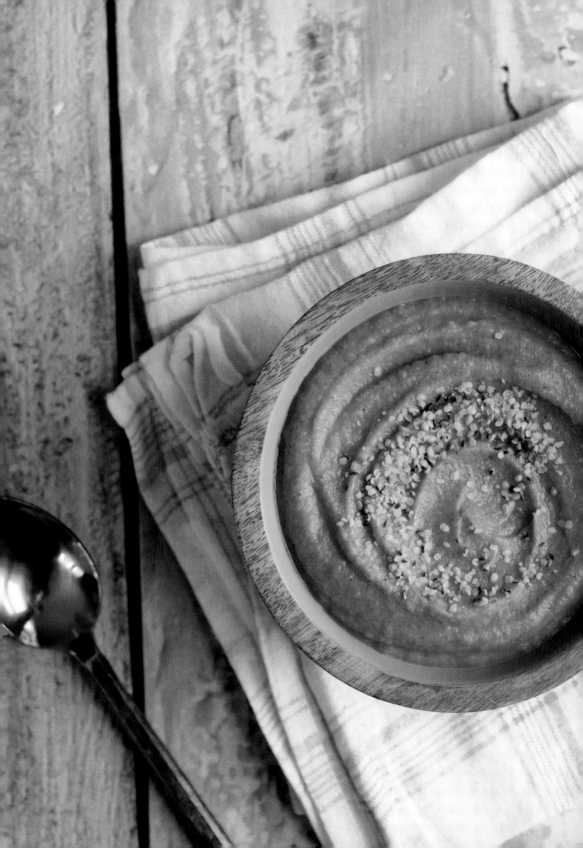

Spicy Butternut Squash Soup

Servings: 4 to 6
1 butternut squash
Olive oil
Salt and pepper, to taste
1 yellow onion, diced
1 large carrot, diced
2 celery stalks, diced
2–3 cloves garlic, minced
2 cups vegetable stock
¼ teaspoon red pepper flakes
½ teaspoon ground sage
1 teaspoon cinnamon
Hemp seeds

1. Preheat oven to 350 degrees.

2. While the oven is preheating, cut the butternut squash in half and place on baking sheet. Drizzle with olive oil, sprinkle salt and pepper, and place it in the oven. Bake for 50–60 minutes or until tender.

3. While the squash is baking, prepare your soup base. In a large sauté pan, drizzle olive oil and heat the onion for 5 minutes or until lightly browned.

4. Add the carrot and celery and continue to sauté for another 10 minutes, mixing occasionally.

5. Add the garlic, salt, and pepper and continue sautéing for another few minutes.

6. Add the vegetable stock, bring to a boil, and then simmer for 35–40 minutes.

7. Add the red pepper flakes, sage, and cinnamon to the mixture.

8. Once the butternut squash is ready, remove and let cool a few minutes.

9. Scoop out the butternut squash, add it to the sauté pan, and stir thoroughly.

10. Put the soup mixture into a high-speed blender and blend until the soup is nice and creamy.

11. Pour into a bowl, top with the hemp seeds, and enjoy!

Note: The soup will be a thicker consistency. If you like a thinner soup, add an additional 1 cup vegetable stock when you blend it.

Also pairs well with the Almond Chia Bread on page 229.

Revamp Wilted Celery or Asparagus!

Nothing stinks more than wilted veggies. After all, that's basically wasted cash and nutrition. But you CAN save some veggies. If your celery or asparagus is starting to wilt, simply cut both ends and stick it in a cup of ice water to help make it nice and crispy again.

Butternut Squash Pasta

Servings: 4 to 6

1 butternut squash, diced

Olive oil

Salt and pepper, to taste

1 yellow onion, diced

3 garlic cloves, minced

1 teaspoon red pepper flakes

1 teaspoon smoked paprika

1 teaspoon sage

1 cup vegetable stock

1 box or bag of your favorite pasta (I love quinoa-and-bean pasta!)

1 cup Swiss chard

1. Preheat oven to 400 degrees.

2. Lightly coat the butternut squash with olive oil, top with salt and pepper, and bake for 30 minutes or until tender.

3. In a large skillet, warm olive oil over medium heat and toss the onions for 5–6 minutes.

4. Add the garlic and toss for 1 minute or until fragrant. Turn off the heat and cover.

5. When the butternut squash is done, place it in the large skillet with the onion, turn up to medium heat, add red pepper flakes, smoked paprika, sage, salt, pepper, and the vegetable stock. Let simmer for about 10 minutes.

6. Prepare the pasta as directed.

7. In a large blender, pour in the butternut squash mixture and blend. Using the same pan, add a little olive oil and toss the Swiss chard for a few minutes or until wilted.

8. Add the butternut squash mixture and pasta to the skillet. Mix generously and season with salt and pepper.

Almond Butter Cup Oats

Servings: 1

½ cup rolled oats
1 cup almond milk
2 tablespoons almond butter
1 tablespoon raw cacao powder
Drizzle of maple syrup
Pinch of sea salt

1. Prepare the rolled oats as directed on the package except substitute 1 cup almond milk for the 1 cup water.

2. Pour the rolled oats in a small bowl and top with the almond butter and raw cacao. Drizzle the maple syrup on top and finish with a pinch of sea salt.

3. You can have an almond butter cup for breakfast or even lunch.

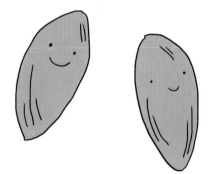

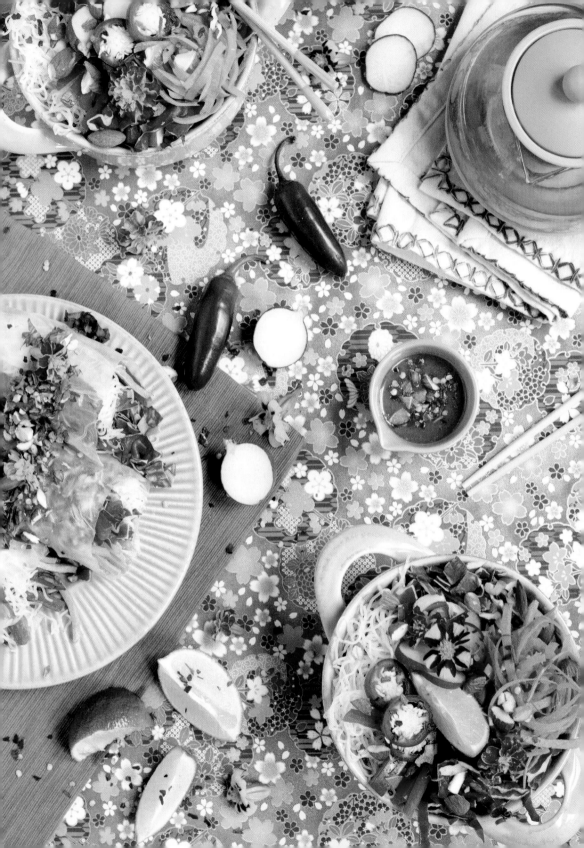

Spring Rolls and Bowls

Spring Rolls with Chili-Almond Dip

Servings: 4

SPRING ROLL INGREDIENTS

4 spring roll rice wrappers
¼ red cabbage head, chopped small
1 red bell pepper, cut into thin strips
1 carrot, cut into thin strips
Cilantro or basil

DIP INGREDIENTS

½ cup almond butter
1 teaspoon sesame oil
1 clove garlic, diced
1-inch piece of ginger, peeled and diced
2 tablespoons liquid amino acids or soy
   sauce
1 tablespoon fresh lime juice
¼ teaspoon crushed red pepper flakes
Crushed almonds, for sprinkling on top

1. Soak the rice wrappers in warm water for 10–20 seconds. Remove and place on a flat surface.

2. Add the cabbage, pepper, carrot, and cilantro or basil. Be careful not to overfill. Flip up the ends of the rice wrapper on both sides and roll up like a burrito.

3. Place the seam side of spring roll on the plate and allow to sit for several minutes to seal.

4. Combine all the dip ingredients in a small bowl, and enjoy with the spring rolls!

Tip: Feel free to add additional vegetables, avocados, thin rice noodles, or other proteins such as tempeh to the spring rolls. These make a great mood-boosting snack and are superfun to eat.

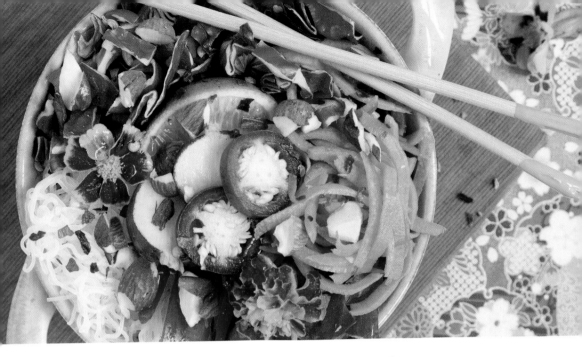

Spring Bowls with Chili-Almond Dressing

Turn your spring rolls inside out with these fun "spring bowls."

Servings: 2

SPRING BOWL INGREDIENTS

½ cup thin rice noodles, cooked
¼ red cabbage head, chopped small
1 red bell pepper, cut into thin strips
1 carrot, cut into thin strips

OPTIONAL TOPPINGS

Jalapeños (if you like additional spice)
Crushed almonds
Cilantro or basil

PROTEIN NOTE: Add tofu or shrimp for an added filling boost.

DRESSING INGREDIENTS

3 tablespoons almond butter
½ teaspoon liquid amino acids
1 tablespoon olive or sesame oil
Pinch of red pepper flakes
¼ teaspoon garlic salt

1. Place all your spring bowl ingredients neatly in a small bowl.

2. Top with the jalapeños, crushed almonds, and cilantro or basil, as desired.

3. Combine all the dressing ingredients in a small bowl, and enjoy with the spring bowls!

EAT YOUR FEELINGS

Spaghetti Squash Bake

Servings: 2
1 spaghetti squash
Olive oil
Salt and pepper, to taste
1 14-ounce jar marinara or 2 6-ounce
  jars pesto sauce
Parmesan cheese (optional)
Pine nuts (optional)

1. Preheat oven to 375 degrees.

2. Cut the spaghetti squash in half and de-seed the inside.

3. Drizzle with olive oil and season with salt and pepper.

4. Place the squash halves with the cut side down in the baking dish. Add a tablespoon or two of water to the baking dish.

5. Roast in the oven for 35–45 minutes or until the squash is tender.

6. Use a fork and scrape out the squash. It will make spaghetti-like strands.

7. From there, mix with either the marinara and Parmesan or the pesto and pine nuts and enjoy!

PROTEIN NOTE: Add a little cooked beef if you want a meatier squash bake. Avoid chicken as it can make you more anxious.

Sweet Potato Chips

Servings: 1 to 2
1 sweet potato, thinly sliced
Olive oil
Sea salt

1. Preheat oven to 225 degrees.

2. Lightly coat the sweet potato slices with olive oil and top with sea salt. Lay them out in a single layer on a baking sheet lined with parchment paper.

3. Bake for about 2 hours, flipping them halfway through.

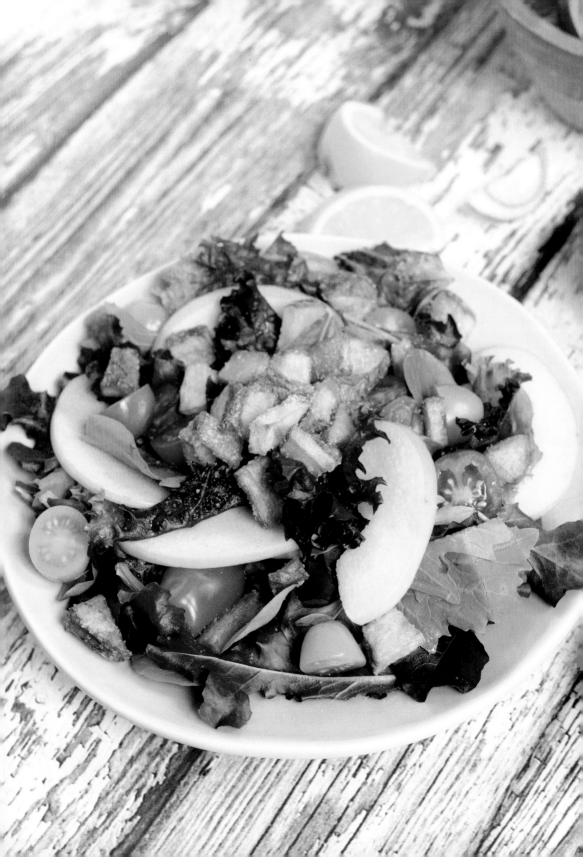

Balsamic Crunch Salad

Servings: 1

1 potato, peeled and cut into small cubes
Olive oil
2 handfuls of spring mix
4 cherry tomatoes, sliced in half
½ pear or apple, sliced thin
Sea salt

1. Preheat oven to 400 degrees.

2. Lightly coat the potato with olive oil and bake for 20–25 minutes or until your desired crispness. (I like mine supercrisp!)

3. Prepare your salad by combining the spring mix, cherry tomatoes, and pear or apple in a medium bowl.

4. Once the potato is done, remove and place in a paper-towel-lined bowl and sprinkle with sea salt.

5. Top the salad off with the potato "croutons" and drizzle with the Easy Breezy Balsamic Dressing.

EASY BREEZY BALSAMIC DRESSING

3 tablespoons olive oil
1 tablespoon balsamic vinegar
Salt and pepper, to toast

Combine all the ingredients in a small bowl or jar. Shake before using.

Tip: If you want to make even more dressing, the ratio is 3 parts oil to 1 part vinegar, so you can make a bigger portion for additional salads during the week.

PROTEIN NOTE: Add a filet of grilled salmon, grilled shrimp, or grilled tofu or tempeh for additional protein to keep you fuller throughout the day.

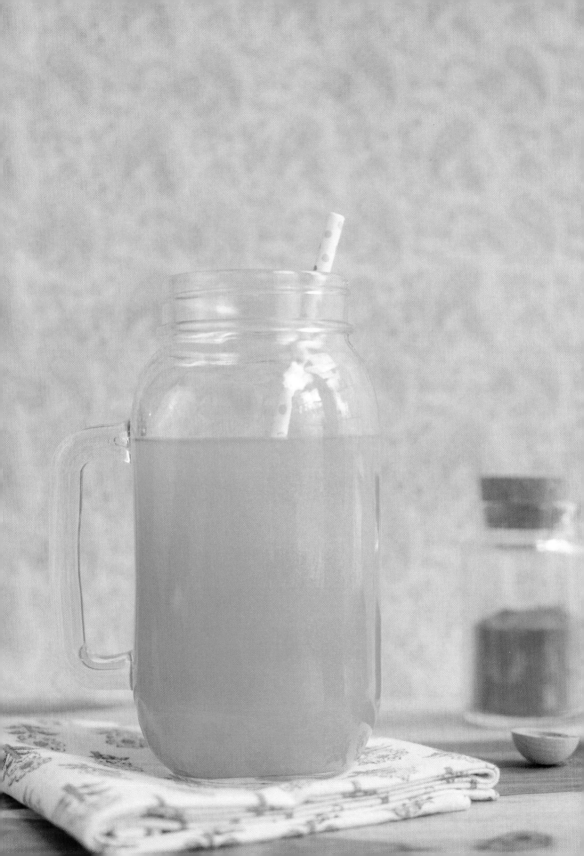

DRINKS

Iced Turmeric Lemonade

Servings: 4
- 1 quart filtered water
- 1 tablespoon turmeric
- 2 lemons, juiced
- 1-2 tablespoons maple syrup (depending on desired sweetness)

1. In a large pitcher, combine the water, turmeric, lemon juice, and maple syrup. Mix until the turmeric is evenly distributed.

2. Pour into a glass and serve with a fun straw!

Turmeric Tonic

Servings: 1
- 1 cup coconut or almond milk
- 1 teaspoon turmeric
- A few thin slices of ginger
- A dash of ground black pepper
- 1 teaspoon maple syrup (optional)

1. Combine all the ingredients in a small saucepan on a low-heat setting.

2. Whisk until the contents are frothy and warm.

3. Pour the contents into a glass and use a cocktail strainer to remove the ginger, if desired.

4. Drink and relax. Wake up refreshed.

Cinnamon Roll Smoothie

Servings: 1
- 1 frozen banana
- 1 cup almond milk
- ½ cup quick oats
- ½ teaspoon cinnamon
- 1 teaspoon pure vanilla extract

Blend all the ingredients and enjoy!

Calming Chamomile Tea

Servings: 1
- 1 teaspoon passionflower
- 1 teaspoon chamomile
- ¼ teaspoon lavender

1. Combine all the ingredients and place in a tea steeper.

2. Steep 5–6 minutes and serve!

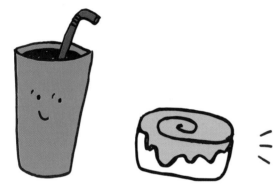

RECIPES

when

YOU'RE FEELING

EXHAUSTED

or

TIRED

EMOTION: EXHAUSTED/TIRED

When we are exhausted and tired, we tend to gravitate toward foods that will provide a quick fix. The last thing you want to do when you are tired is actually think about cooking or making something.

However, the more you turn to things like caffeine and sugar to overcome your exhaustion, the more those things wreak havoc on your body, and eventually those quick fixes don't work anymore.

The goal is to fuel your body with foods during the day that will naturally keep your energy high as opposed to choosing quick fixes that will leave you feeling good temporarily but then crashing even harder.

In this section, you will find foods that you can start incorporating into your daily life that will help lift your energy naturally. And while there are some "quick fix" recipes that you can use for an instant boost, most are designed to keep your energy levels steady rather than give you a boost and then crash later.

Plus, you can still have your coffee and drink it, too.

SIGNS AND SYMPTOMS OF TIRED EATING

- You are yawning while trying to drink your vanilla latte.
- You doze off during a training session and attempt to wake yourself up by eating all the free candies on the table.
- Coffee stops giving you the energy boost you crave.
- The second you get home at night, making food suddenly feels like the hardest thing to do ever.
- You snack on things when you aren't even hungry in hopes it will keep you awake.
- You crave high-fat, high-carb foods.

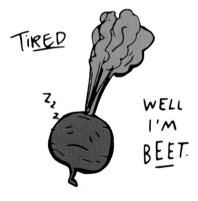

TIRED

WELL I'M BEET.

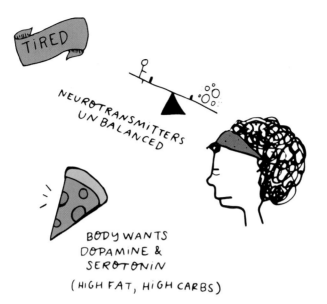

TIRED

NEUROTRANSMITTERS UNBALANCED

BODY WANTS DOPAMINE & SEROTONIN
(HIGH FAT, HIGH CARBS)

WHAT'S (REALLY) HAPPENING TO YOUR BODY?

Being tired all the time is not normal.

In our fast-paced society, it's easy to get caught up in the hustle of life. Life is basically one superlong to-do list. There is always something to add on or check off, and it's easy to spend a majority of the time worrying about all the tasks rather than completing them.

For many people, physical exhaustion is a badge of honor. It helps them feel as if they are making a difference or they are successful. After all, if you're exhausted, it means you are working hard. Unfortunately, physical exhaustion is not something worth achieving because it has short-term and long-term consequences that can't be fixed by a job promotion or a pat on the back.

When you overwork yourself and your body becomes physically exhausted, you get sick faster, gain weight more easily, and can develop major mood issues such as anxiety and depression.

You might also find yourself craving foods high in fat and carbohydrates— except rather than eating a quinoa-and-avocado salad, you opt for pizza and breadsticks. When you are exhausted, your body's neurotransmitters are out of balance. In order to seek balance, your body seeks out dopamine and serotonin, which can be found in high-fat and high-carb foods. Most of the time, we grab junk food, which only keeps the exhaustion train riding even farther, leaving you feeling depressed, lethargic, and unable to fall asleep.

BEST FOODS KNOWN TO BOOST ENERGY

Apples
Avocados
Bananas
Berries
Broccoli
Brussels sprouts
Dark leafy greens
Ginger
Grass-fed meats
Kohlrabi
Limes
Mangoes
Matcha
Nuts and seeds
Olives
Pineapples
Quinoa
Water
Lemons

Why These Foods?

Water: Proper hydration is essential for energy. Oftentimes, we try to sneak a quick caffeine boost when in reality our body just needs some good old H_2O—or, as my husband would say, "Water: the original energy drink."

Electrolytes: Consuming foods or drinks with electrolytes can help your cells get the energy they need to keep you moving.

Vitamin C: Foods high in vitamin C help turn fat into energy, giving your body a quick boost.

Fiber: Foods high in fiber can help balance blood sugar levels to keep your energy stable throughout the day.

B Vitamins: These vitamins help turn carbohydrates into glucose, which can help you go from food to fuel really fast.

Iron: Low iron can often result in chronic fatigue, light-headedness, dizziness, and overall body weakness. Ensuring you have enough iron is crucial for maintaining a high level of sustainable energy.

Healthy Fat: No, eating fat does not make you fat. In fact, eating healthy fat can help keep your brain functioning and your energy levels high. Since most of your brain is made up of fat, it needs fat in order to think clearly and function at the highest capacity.

EAT YOUR FEELINGS

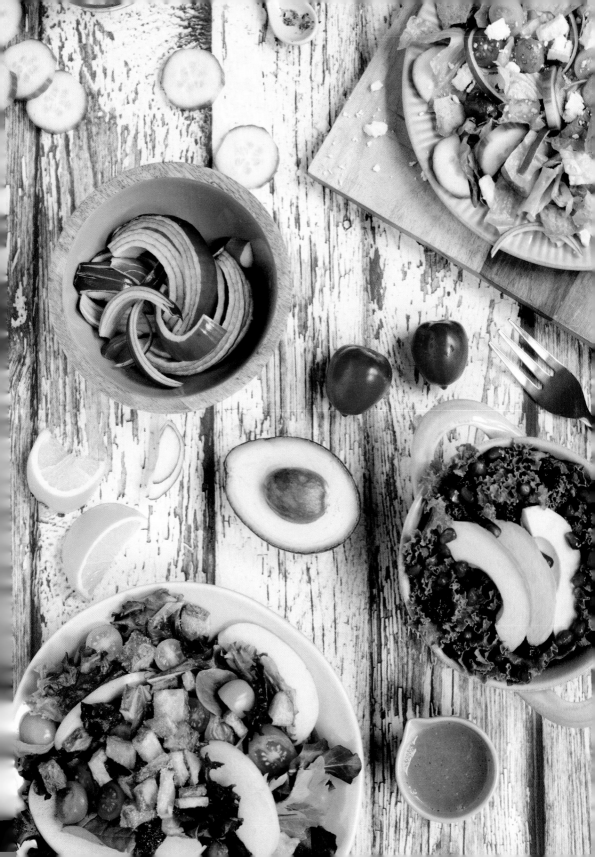

OTHER TYPES OF FOODS TO EAT

Spicy Foods: Spicy foods in general tend to awaken your senses and give your body a nice energy boost.

Fermented Foods: Since fermented foods naturally contain probiotics, they are easy on the gut and therefore easy to digest. The less energy your body has to spend digesting food, the more energy you get to be a human! (Ever wonder why you feel lethargic after Thanksgiving? All those meats and carbs take a long time to digest, making you feel sluggish!)

LIFESTYLE "FOODS"

- Get plenty of rest. Sleep is a "superfood," so plan on getting to bed early for a few nights in a row. Shut down your cell phone and other electronic devices an hour before you go to bed.
- Make a to-don't list. List all the things you are going to commit to NOT doing if someone asks you. Make yourself a priority!
- Stretch. Do some simple cat and cow stretches or a downward dog to get some energy moving in your body. It doesn't have to be hard—think simple!
- Drink water. Oftentimes when we feel fatigued, our body is really dehydrated. Try drinking some water to reenergize. Add some lemon for an additional refreshing boost.
- Get out in the sunshine. A few minutes in the sun is enough to increase your energy and your mood. Whether it means just sitting outside for a few minutes or going on a quick walk, sunshine can do wonders for your body and soul.

SWEET

Easy Energy Bars

Servings: 12 to 16

½ cup raw cashews, chopped
½ cup raw almonds, chopped
½ cup raw peanuts, chopped
½ cup sunflower seeds, chopped
½ cup peanut butter or almond butter, melted
⅓ cup brown rice syrup or raw or local honey, melted

1. Line an 8-inch-square pan with parchment paper or waxed paper.

2. In a medium bowl, combine the cashews, almonds, peanuts, and sunflower seeds. Slowly add the peanut or almond butter and rice syrup or honey. Stir until the mixture forms one solid ball.

3. Press into the prepared pan. Refrigerate for 60 minutes, then cut into 12 squares. Wrap individual bars in plastic wrap or store in an airtight container and refrigerate.

Happy Quinoa Bowl

Servings: 1

½ cup cooked quinoa (warm)
1 teaspoon ground cinnamon
2 tablespoons almond butter
¼ cup fresh blueberries
Raw or local honey
Almond milk

1. In a small bowl, mix the warm quinoa with the cinnamon and almond butter.

2. Top with the blueberries, then add the honey and almond milk to taste.

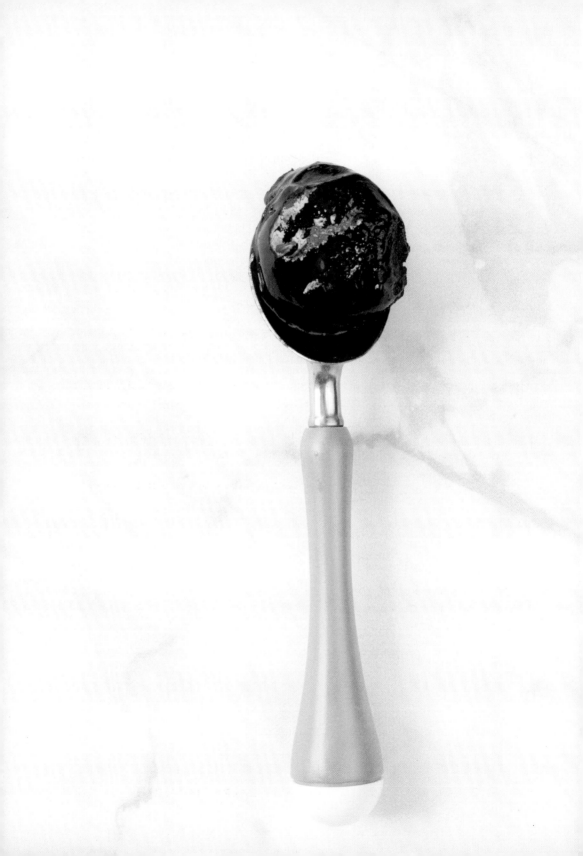

Charcoal Ice Cream

Servings: 2
- 1 cup nut milk
- 1 teaspoon charcoal powder
- 1 teaspoon grated fresh ginger
- 1 lemon, juiced
- 1 tablespoon maple syrup (or more for desired sweetness)

1. Place all the ingredients in an ice cream maker as directed.

2. Enjoy this ice cream the next time you have a stomachache or want something to cool down.

Activated Charcoal to Ease Stomach Pains (and Whiten Teeth)

If you are traveling and eating out at various restaurants, pack some activated charcoal for your trip to prevent stomach issues. It absorbs bad bacteria and can leave your stomach feeling relaxed. Bonus: You can also brush your teeth with it and it will help naturally whiten them!

Tea Cookies

Servings: 12 to 14
- 2 cups flour (I used gluten-free cup for cup)
- 2 tablespoons Earl Grey tea (you can also use chamomile, green, or your favorite loose-leaf tea)
- Pinch of salt
- Zest from 1 lemon
- 1 cup coconut oil
- ½ cup honey
- ½ teaspoon pure vanilla extract

1. In a large bowl, combine all the dry ingredients and mix.

2. Add all the liquid ingredients and mix until a ball starts to form.

3. Refrigerate for 30 minutes. Preheat oven to 350 degrees.

4. Roll and cut out cookies in your favorite shape.

5. Bake for 12–14 minutes.

6. Let the cookies cool completely before serving.

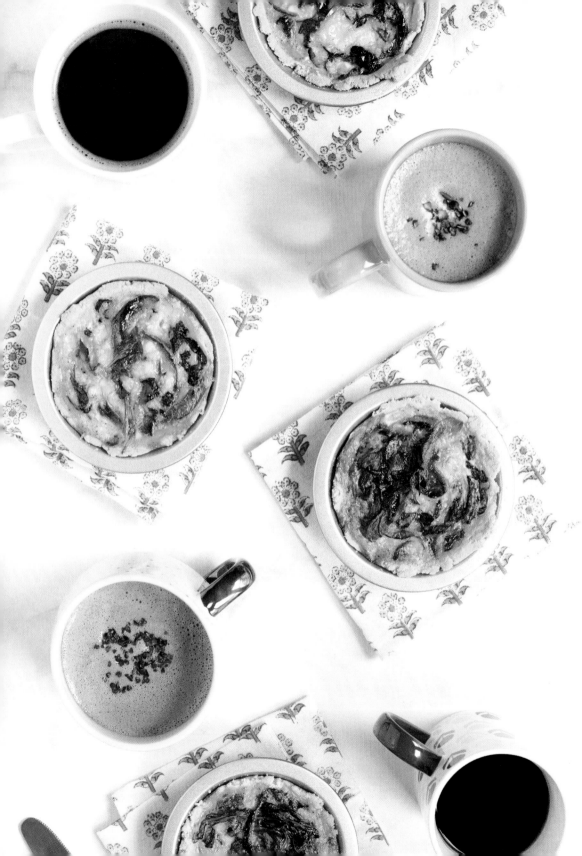

Mini Quiches

Servings: 4

ALMOND-PARMESAN CRUST INGREDIENTS

1½ cups almond meal
½ cup Parmesan cheese
1 teaspoon baking powder
1 egg
1 tablespoon olive oil
4 mini pie pans

1. Combine all the ingredients in a medium bowl and mix until it gets lumpy. Then use your hands to form one solid dough ball.

2. Break the dough into four equal parts and press them in the four mini pie pans. Place in the refrigerator until ready to use.

FILLING INGREDIENTS

Olive oil
½ yellow onion, diced
½ red pepper, diced
2 bunches of kale, de-stemmed and chopped
Salt and pepper, to taste
4 eggs
⅓ cup Gouda cheese, shredded

1. In a medium skillet coated with olive oil on medium heat, sauté the onion for about 5 minutes or until lightly browned.

2. Add the red pepper and sauté for an additional 5 minutes.

3. Add the kale and cook until wilted. Season the dish with salt and pepper. Remove from the heat.

4. In a mixing bowl, whisk your eggs. Add the sautéed vegetables and the cheese, mix, and pour into the mini pie pans, making sure the egg mixture doesn't rise above the crust.

5. Bake for 15–20 minutes or until golden brown on top.

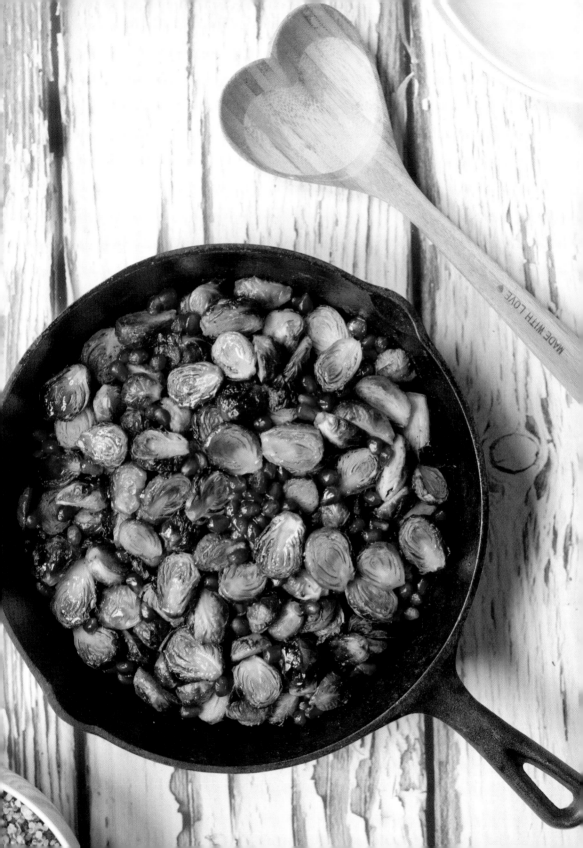

Made-with-Love Brussels

Servings: 4 to 6
2 cups Brussels sprouts
Olive oil
Salt and pepper, to taste
½ cup pomegranate seeds
Balsamic vinegar

1. Preheat oven to 350 degrees.

2. Cut the Brussels sprouts in half and place in a medium bowl.

3. Drizzle with balsamic vinegar and olive oil and mix until it's evenly distributed. Season with salt and pepper.

4. Place your Brussel sprouts in a cast-iron baking dish or on a baking sheet, and bake for 25–30 minutes or until they are crisp.

5. Remove from the heat and let cool for about 5 minutes, then top with the pomegranate seeds and serve!

EAT WITH LOVE

Kale? Love it up!

Cupcakes? Feel the joy!

Whether it's kale or a cupcake, go into every eating experience with a sense of love and gratitude.

Stop to appreciate everything the experience of eating that food is bringing you. Think about how the ingredients got to your plate, how the chef prepared it with love, and feel a sense of joy for the nourishment it's providing you.

Many times, we feel so ashamed about what we are consuming that we end up berating ourselves for wanting or eating something we think of as "bad." Other times, we eat mindlessly, in haste, barely acknowledging hunger or satiation. When we put negative energy and emotion into our food, this energy shows up in our bodies as negative moods, low energy, and low self-esteem.

So the next time you go to eat, whether it's fast food, convenience food, or farm-fresh food, enter each relationship with food with a sense of love, gratitude, and appreciation. Not only will you digest your food better, but you will feel better about eating it. This will result in long-term food love rather than long-term food guilt.

Stuffed Peppers

Servings: 4

1 small + 4 large green bell peppers
1 tablespoon olive oil
3 garlic cloves, crushed
1 onion, chopped
1½ cups cooked quinoa
1 16-ounce can stewed or chunk tomatoes
1 15-ounce can chickpeas
Sea salt and ground black pepper

1. Preheat oven to 350 degrees.

2. Cut off the tops of the large bell peppers. Scoop out the seeds and pithy membrane, taking care not to puncture the skin. Set the hollowed-out peppers aside. Chop the small bell pepper and the large pepper tops, discarding the stems.

3. Heat the olive oil in a large skillet over medium heat. Add the chopped bell pepper, garlic, and onion, and cook for about 3 minutes or until softened. Remove from the heat and mix in the quinoa, tomatoes, and chickpeas.

4. Fill the hollowed-out bell peppers with the quinoa mixture. Place them upright in an oven pan or casserole dish. Pour ½ inch of water into the pan to help them steam; then cover with foil and bake for 45 minutes or until the peppers are soft. Season with salt and pepper to taste.

PROTEIN NOTE: Add a little cooked beef or chicken if you want a meatier stuffed pepper.

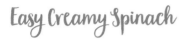

CREAMY

Easy Creamy Spinach

Servings: 2
- 1 package frozen spinach
- 1-2 tablespoons butter
- ½ tablespoon apple cider vinegar
- Salt and pepper, to taste
- Hemp seeds, to taste

1. Boil water in a medium saucepan, add spinach, and reduce the heat. Heat for 5–7 minutes or until the spinach becomes soft. Remove the spinach from the water.

2. In a large blender, combine the spinach, butter, apple cider vinegar, and salt and pepper. Blend until smooth and creamy.

3. Sprinkle some hemp seeds on top and enjoy!

Order a Side of Greens

When you are eating out, always order a side of sautéed greens. This will help give you an energy boost, keep you more regular, and ensure that you are getting some daily veggies.

Chovocado Mousse

Servings: 2
- 1 avocado
- 1 banana (preferably frozen)
- ½ cup almond or rice milk
- 1 tablespoon raw cacao powder
- ½ tablespoon honey or maple syrup (or more if you like it sweet!)
- Ice cubes (if desired)

1. In a blender, combine the avocado, banana, almond or rice milk, raw cacao, and honey or maple syrup until smooth. Add the ice for a thicker texture, if desired.

2. Serve immediately.

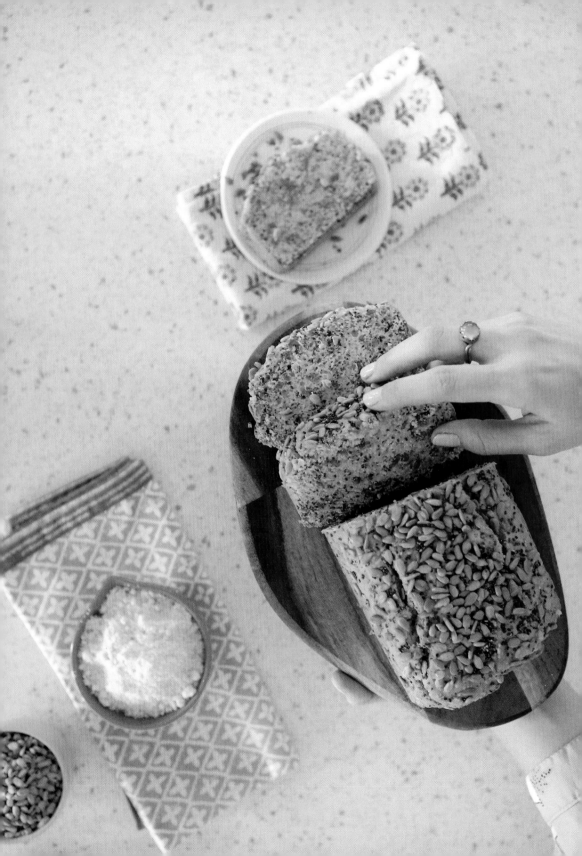

Tomato Soup with Grilled Cheese Croutons

Servings: 6 to 8
  15 plum tomatoes, cut in half lengthwise
  Olive oil
  Salt and pepper, to taste
  1 large yellow onion, diced
  8 garlic cloves, minced
  ¼ teaspoon red pepper flakes
  1 28-ounce can plum tomatoes, with juice
  3 packages (⅔ ounces each) basil leaves
  1 quart vegetable stock

1. Preheat oven to 400 degrees.

2. On a large baking sheet, lay out the plum tomatoes, drizzle with olive oil, and season with salt and pepper. Roast for about 45 minutes.

3. In a large pot on medium heat, add olive oil and sauté the onion for 2–3 minutes. Add the garlic and red pepper flakes and cook for an additional 7–8 minutes or until the onion starts to brown.

4. Add the canned tomatoes, basil, and vegetable stock.

5. When the tomatoes are done roasting, add them to the pot with any extra liquid.

6. Season with salt and pepper, bring to a boil, reduce the heat to low, then let simmer for 30–40 minutes.

7. Remove from the heat and transfer the soup to a high-powered blender and blend until smooth. Sprinkle Grilled Cheese Croutons on top and serve immediately.

GRILLED CHEESE CROUTONS

  4 slices bread (your choice)
  2 tablespoons unsalted butter
  4 ounces Gruyère cheese, shredded

1. Butter one side of each bread slice.

2. Turn two slices over and sprinkle the Gruyère on the unbuttered side.

3. Place the remaining slices of bread on top of the Gruyère, butter side up.

4. In a medium pan, grill the sandwiches for about 4 minutes on each side or until browned.

5. Cut into small cubes and sprinkle on top of the tomato soup!

Note: You also can use a panini press to make the croutons!
   For a healthier twist, use the Almond Chia Bread on page 229. Simply add a little butter, top with cheese, and toast in a toaster oven until desired crispness.

Broccoli + Cheddar Sweet Potato Boats

Servings: 2
1 broccoli head, chopped in small pieces
Olive oil
Sea salt and pepper, to taste
2 sweet potatoes, cut in half lengthwise
2 tablespoons Greek yogurt
¼ cup cheddar cheese

1. Preheat oven to 350 degrees.

2. Put the broccoli on a large baking sheet and drizzle with olive oil, then toss until covered. Sprinkle with sea salt. Coat the flat part of the sweet potatoes with olive oil and turn them flat-side down on the baking sheet.

3. Bake the broccoli for 15–20 minutes or until as crispy as desired, then remove from the baking sheet and set aside.

4. Bake the sweet potatoes for an additional 10–15 minutes or until cooked through.

5. Once the sweet potatoes are done, let them cool for about 10 minutes. Then scoop out the flesh and set the skins back on the baking sheet.

6. In a food processor, blend the sweet potato flesh with the yogurt, sea salt, and pepper.

7. Once the mixture is smooth and creamy, add the broccoli and mix in by hand.

8. Put the sweet potato filling in each of the potato skins, top with the cheddar cheese, and bake for 7–8 minutes or until the cheese is fully melted.

9. Serve as an appetizer or make as a fun midday snack on the weekend!

Slow Applesauce

Servings: 8 to 12
12-15 apples (I use a basket of mixed apples)
1 cup water
2 tablespoons fresh lemon juice (1 small lemon)
3 teaspoons ground cinnamon
Ground cloves, ground nutmeg, and cinnamon stick (optional)

1. Peel, core, and cube the apples.

2. Place in a slow cooker with the water and lemon juice. Add the ground cinnamon and the cloves, nutmeg, and cinnamon stick, if desired. Stir everything together. Cover.

3. Cook on low for 4–6 hours, checking the consistency every ½ hour after the fourth hour. To thicken the applesauce, cook with the lid off for the last ½ hour.

4. Remove the cinnamon stick, if used. With a whisk or an immersion blender, mix the applesauce well. Serve warm or cold.

"I Woke Up Like This"

Do you wake up each morning feeling flawless or like a grumpy monster that doesn't even know what day it is?

Sleep is an underrated yet powerful "nutrient" when it comes to creating a healthy lifestyle. It is truly one of the most powerful healing mechanisms we have.

Each night, while your body is asleep, an internal cleaning crew cleanses your insides to prep your body for the following day. It helps rebalance your hormones, detox your cells, and recharge your body. A lack of sleep delays this process, and over time, your body breaks down.

We have to shift from thinking of sleep as a luxury to understanding it as an essential part of living. Think of sleep as a vital nutrient or a superfood that can greatly impact your overall health and well-being.

Here are some ways to catch more zzz's and wake up flawless every day:

1. **Turn down the lights.** Turn off your electronics at least an hour before you head to bed. This will help wind down your brain, relax your eyes, and prepare your body for a good night's sleep.
2. **Get rid of things that make you uncomfortable.** For some people, any little light entering the room can trigger their senses and keep them awake. Try using light-blocking curtains and putting tape on little electronics that have red or green dots that can cause disturbances. Additionally, if you have a messy room or things are out of order, this may inhibit your sleeping as well. Set your room up as a comfortable oasis so you can ensure you get the best night's sleep possible.
3. **Allow yourself time to wind down.** Oftentimes, we head to bed after we've exhausted all other forms of entertainment. However, give yourself some time to wind down from the day. This includes activities, TV, phone, friends, or work. Try to go to your bed 30 minutes before you are ready to fall asleep so you can give yourself some time to wind down and relax.
4. **Nap when necessary.** Ever experience a midday headache? You may think it's dehydration or stress, but it could also be lack of sleep. The better the sleep I get, the more I notice when my body has not had enough. When a headache comes on, I immediately recognize that lack of sleep is the culprit and I know just how to fix it: a nap. If you feel run-down and tired, a quick fifteen-minute nap might be enough to get you re-energized for the day.

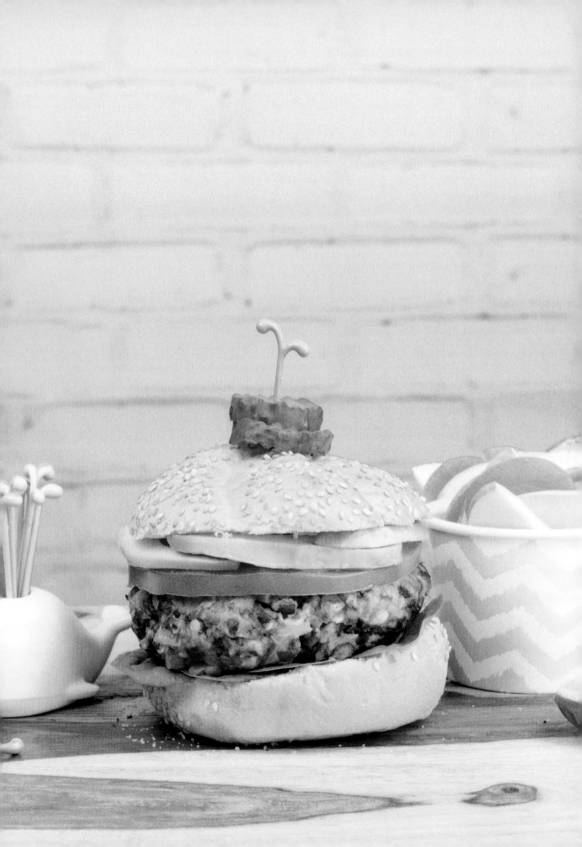

CRUNCHY

Black Bean Burger + Kohlrabi Slaw

Servings: 4 to 6
  2 tablespoons olive oil
  1 small red onion, diced
  1 clove garlic, minced
  1 red pepper, diced small
  1 15-ounce can black beans, rinsed
    and drained
  1 tablespoon sesame oil
  1 teaspoon chipotle powder or chili powder
  1 teaspoon cumin
  Salt and pepper, to taste
  ½ cup quick-cooking oats
  ½ cup quinoa
  1 egg

1. In a skillet over medium heat, warm the olive oil. Add the onion, garlic, and red pepper and cook for 5–10 minutes or until softened.

2. Transfer the vegetables to a blender or food processor and set the skillet aside. Add the black beans, sesame oil, spices, and salt and pepper and pulse until combined but still chunky. Pulse in the oats, quinoa, and egg. Form the mixture into patties.

3. In the skillet, add more oil if necessary and cook the patties over medium heat

for 2–3 minutes or until golden brown. Flip and brown the other side.

4. Enjoy on buns or go topless and add extra veggies!

KOHLRABI SLAW

Servings: 2 to 4
  2 large carrots, thinly sliced
  1 turnip, thinly sliced
  1 kohlrabi, thinly sliced

LEMON-TAHINI DRESSING

  ¼ cup tahini
  1 lemon, juiced
  3-5 tablespoons warm water
  1-2 garlic cloves, minced
  Salt and pepper, to taste

1. Combine all the vegetables in a bowl and toss to mix.

2. To prepare the dressing, combine ingredients in a blender and blend for 30 seconds.

3. Serve the dressing on the side or toss on the vegetables and serve.

Go-To Quinoa Salad

Servings: 6 to 8
  1 cup dry quinoa, rinsed well
  ½ cup pine nuts
  ¼ cup olive oil + additional for the skillet
  1 tablespoon maple syrup
  ¼ cup lemon juice
  ½ cup diced red bell peppers
  ½ cup diced red onion
  1 bunch parsley, chopped
  1 cucumber, diced
  ½ cup dried cranberries
  Sea salt and ground black pepper

1. Cook the quinoa according to the package directions. Let cool.

2. In a small skillet, toast the pine nuts with a little olive oil on low heat for 5–10 minutes.

3. In a small bowl, whisk together ¼ cup olive oil, maple syrup, lemon juice, and salt and black pepper to taste.

4. In a large bowl, combine the quinoa, bell peppers, onion, parsley, cucumber, and cranberries. Top with the pine nuts, then drizzle with the dressing. Toss and enjoy!

PROTEIN NOTE: Add a little shrimp or canned salmon for an additional protein boost.

Kale Chips

Servings: 1 to 2
  3 bunches kale, stems removed
  1–2 tablespoons olive oil
  2 pinches of sea salt

1. Preheat the oven to 325 degrees.

2. Spread the kale on a baking sheet. Place the oil in a bowl, dip your fingers, and rub a very light coating over the kale. Sprinkle on the sea salt.

3. Bake for 7–12 minutes, turning the kale halfway through the cooking time, until it turns a bit brown. Watch carefully because it can burn quickly.

MOOD-ENHANCING ADD-ONS

Nutritional yeast + cashews for a cheesy flavor
Chipotle seasoning to give it a kick
Garlic salt and/or minced garlic to fight off vampires

EAT YOUR FEELINGS

Eat Kale, but Don't Be a D*ck

"You can eat as much kale as humanly possible and you can still be a dick. No amount of leafy greens will make you a kind person." —Confucius

Just kidding, I said this.

Food shaming in the health industry is a growing problem as more and more people become conscious of their food choices.

I find that people who know a ton about health and nutrition can sometimes come across with a tinge of superiority, thinking that their way is the only way. Why do you think there are so many health and diet books claiming to be the end-all, cure-all for everything, yet all of them contradict one another?

As a food-mood-etarian, I personally do not follow any sort of rules or regimens when it comes to healthy living and eating. I often experiment with my body to figure out what works for me, and I check in often because it changes over time.

I remember one night I posted a picture of a frozen pizza and broccoli I was eating for dinner. Granted, this isn't my everyday food choice, but sometimes a girl just wants a frozen pizza and some broccoli.

Immediately after posting, the food shamers started coming to the surface and flipped out on me for posting a picture of a slice of pizza. My first thought was "But it's gluten-free and organic. Doesn't that count for something?" My second thought was "Am I a fraud? Am I a bad person?" And my third thought, well, I'll leave that to your imagination.

But that's when I realized that food holds such emotional value for us. We have deep beliefs around food, and oftentimes if we see a change in ourselves, we turn into food evangelicals who want to preach the way to healthy salvation. And while I can appreciate the enthusiasm and deep commitment, oftentimes it turns people from a place of love to a place of fear, and they end up food shaming and making others feel bad rather than appreciating others for their unique journey.

So let's eat our kale, eat our pizza, and remember to be kind throughout it all. Everyone has a different journey when it comes to food, so let's be kind, meet people where they are, listen deeply, and, in general, don't be a dick.

Simple Bean Salad

Servings: 4 to 6

SALAD INGREDIENTS

1 15-ounce can chickpeas, drained and rinsed
1 15-ounce can red beans, drained and rinsed
2 carrots, chopped
½ onion, chopped
1 red pepper, chopped

DRESSING INGREDIENTS

¼ cup olive oil
8 tablespoons balsamic vinegar
¼ cup cilantro, chopped
1 tablespoon raw honey
A few dashes of cumin, to taste
Salt and pepper, to taste

1. To make the salad, combine the beans in a medium-size the bowl.

2. Add the carrots, onion, and red pepper.

3. To make the dressing, combine the dressing ingredients in a separate bowl.

4. Pour the dressing over the salad mixture and stir.

5. Enjoy immediately, or chill for a few hours to let the flavors soak in.

PROTEIN NOTE: You can use any beans you have on hand.

DRINKS

Matcha Latte

Servings: 1
8 ounces almond or coconut milk
1 teaspoon matcha powder
Maple syrup or honey

1. In a small saucepan, bring the almond or coconut milk to a low simmer.

2. In a coffee mug, place the matcha and slowly add the milk. Use a mini whisk to froth up the milk and mix in the matcha.

3. Add maple syrup or honey, depending on your desired level of sweetness.

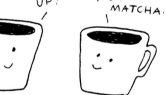

No-Jitters Java

Servings: 1
  8 ounces hot coffee
  1 tablespoon grass-fed butter or coconut oil
  1 teaspoon raw cacao powder
  1 teaspoon maple syrup
  ½ teaspoon reishi mushroom powder
    (optional)

1. Combine all the ingredients in a blender and blend until smooth and frothy.

2. Drink and unleash your energized power!

Berry Burst Smoothie

Servings: 1
  ¼ cup frozen blueberries
  ¼ cup frozen cherries
  ½ banana
  Handful of spinach
  1 cup almond milk

1. Blend all ingredients and serve immediately

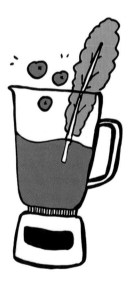

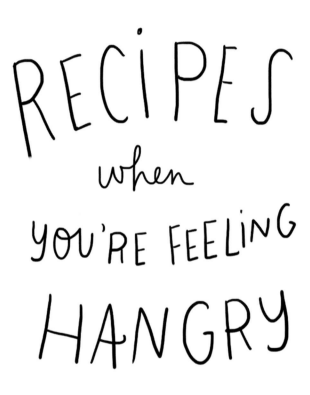

RECIPES
when
YOU'RE FEELING
HANGRY

EMOTION: HANGRY

Don't let the hanger pangs fool you. Hanger can strike at any time, day or night. It can happen in the car, at work, after a long day . . . when you least expect it.

Aside from the emotional outburst over whether your significant other did the laundry (for their sake, please hope the answer is yes, yes, they did the laundry), hanger can affect everything from your food choices to your hormones.

When canned meat starts looking like food porn or you find yourself crying into a bag of chips, you know the force of hanger is upon you. You don't care whether it was made by Julia Child or a child. You just need food and you need it now.

According to a survey conducted by the Harris Poll, more than half of Americans admit to being hangry or witnessing others in a hanger episode. That means, statistically, you are more likely to be involved in a hanger incident than you are to vote in a local election or have a savings account. That's a lot of people crying into bags of chips or directing outbursts at loved ones.

While often undiagnosed, hanger is a real issue that can take a toll on your health. Whether you sometimes accidentally forget to eat or make it a daily habit, the long-term effects can lead you to feeling agitated, angry, and moody toward others and yourself on a daily basis.

It's important to ensure you are prepared, eat throughout the day, and use your snack attack station to alleviate any hanger pangs and give your body the proper nutrition it deserves.

In this section, you will find that most of the recipes are supersimple because when you're hangry, the last thing you want to do is look and shop for a million ingredients. Many recipes also have sustaining superpowers, which means they will keep you fuller for longer to keep your hanger pangs at bay.

LS

☑ BREAKFAST- COFFEE!

☑ LUNCH- SALAD!

☑ SNACK - APPLE!

☑ DINNER- BROCCOLI !

☑ HANGRY!!

SIGNS AND SYMPTOMS OF HANGER

- You hear "monster grumbles" in your stomach, or a "Symphony of Gurgling."
- Your mouth is watering. (Even objects like tables and humans look appealing.)
- Processed, packaged foods look like straight-up food porn.
- You call people out for no reason. ("Hey, you! Yeah, I'm talking to you!")
- You experience fits of rage.
- You dissolve into tears for no reason. (You are often found crying into a bag of chips.)
- You get the hunger shakes. (Did someone just say "shake"?! Do you have cookie dough?)
- You have an extra-large headache (with fries).
- Your muscles feel weak (no matter how hard you hit the gym).

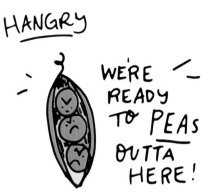

WHAT'S (REALLY) HAPPENING TO YOUR BODY?

Food is made up of a mix of carbohydrates, proteins, and fats. All of these are essential for a healthy diet and a good attitude. Once food is ingested, your system breaks it down into a simple sugar, which is a mix of glucose, amino acids, and fatty acids. Glucose is absorbed in the stomach and the small intestine and eventually released into your bloodstream for steady energy throughout the day. Amino acids are the building blocks of health and help keep your organs functioning. They also help transport and store nutrients in your body. Lastly, fatty acids are crucial because they not only are absorbed in the bloodstream, but they also store energy. So if glucose is very low, the body will use these fatty acids to ensure you are energized and ready to go.

IN A HURRY,
TINY BREAKFAST
(LOW GLUCOSE)

— FIGHT-OR-FLIGHT

— HORMONES GO NUTS
TRYING TO GIVE
YOUR BODY ENERGY

HANGER SHAKES

Combined, these nutrients make their way through your bloodstream and give life force to all your organs, from your brain to your heart to your liver. The result is a happy, healthy, and hanger-free attitude.

But let's say instead of a healthy breakfast full of carbohydrates, proteins, and fats, you opt for a small bowl of cereal or a granola bar, or even nothing at all. Little or no food triggers the fight-or-flight mode in your body. Your body is tricked into thinking that you are in a life-threatening situation in which you might starve to death. Little does it know you were running late because you just had to get on Facebook, or you used your last egg in the brownie mix the night before so there went breakfast. Instead,

your body wants to protect you and keep you alive as long as possible.

In order to do that, your hormones go crazy. Adrenaline and cortisol, both of which are released by the adrenal glands, start to fire off to give your body the energy it needs to sustain itself without food. Your body is attempting to compensate for the low glucose levels. You may also start to get brain fog or the hanger shakes because your body can only keep producing these energy-inducing hormones for so long before you start to crash.

Please note: Hanger shake is not a new milkshake at your local Dairy Queen.

BEST FOODS KNOWN TO FIGHT OFF HANGER

Almonds

Apples

Artichokes

Avocados

Bananas

Beans

Carrots

Cauliflower

Chia seeds

Collard greens

Eggs

Onions

Pears

Quinoa

Radicchio

Rutabagas

Water

Why These Foods?

When you're hangry, your blood sugar is typically low, which is why it's important to fuel up with snacks that are categorized as complex carbohydrates. They will give you the boost of blood sugar you need without the crash.

Fiber: Fiber helps slow down sugar absorption, which can help keep your blood sugar stabilized throughout the day. Fiber can also help keep your digestive tract moving, which can help eliminate toxins and keep your body healthy and happy.

Chromium: This mineral helps your body metabolize carbohydrates and fat. This can help control your blood sugar levels so you aren't left yelling at your significant other because the toilet paper roll is the wrong way. (Come on, we all know it's supposed to go over.)

Magnesium: Aside from helping with your brain function, magnesium can also help stabilize blood sugar levels. And seeing as nearly 75 percent of Americans are magnesium deficient, it's important to ensure you are eating magnesium-rich foods.

OTHER TYPES OF FOODS TO EAT

Filling Foods: To avoid being hangry in the future, eat items that will keep you fuller for longer, such as healthy fats like avocado and nuts, healthy carbohydrates such as quinoa, and protein such as eggs and tempeh.

Cooked Foods: If you graze throughout the day, chances are you are eating mainly processed foods or raw snacks. Cooked foods give your body a warming sensation, help with the digestion process, and make you feel like you actually ate a meal rather than just grazed. This can help you feel fuller longer and genuinely more satisfied.

LIFESTYLE "FOODS"

- Use the snack attack station on page 84 to create stations at home and in the car to have snacks on hand that you can eat to avoid being hangry.
- Shop when full. Eat a snack before you head to the grocery store, or shop after dinner. When you're grocery shopping while hangry, not only do you feel irritable, but you end up buying $100 worth of easy snacks that you will regret eating later on.
- Engage your brain. If you are going to be without food for a while, find an activity to keep you occupied and keep the hanger pangs at bay. Play a fun game on your phone or do a crossword puzzle.

Chunky Monkey Banana Bites

Servings: 1
  1 banana
  Nut butter (your choice)
  Dark chocolate chips

1. Slice the banana into ½-inch coins.

2. Place one coin down and add a small scoop of nut butter on top.

3. Sprinkle a few chocolate chips on top.

4. Place another banana slice on top of the nut butter and chocolate chips. It will look like a little mini sandwich.

5. Enjoy!

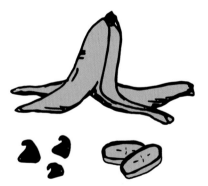

Mini Blueberry Muffins

Servings: 18 to 24
  2 cups almond flour
  1½ teaspoons baking soda
  ½ teaspoon sea salt
  ¼ cup maple syrup
  ¼ cup applesauce
  2 tablespoons coconut oil
  1 teaspoon pure vanilla extract
  1 cup blueberries

1. Preheat oven to 350 degrees.

2. Combine all the ingredients except the blueberries in a food processor. Blend until smooth.

3. In a large bowl, fold the blueberries into the batter.

4. Grease or line a mini muffin pan or use a silicone muffin mold (my fav!), and drop in the batter a tablespoon at a time.

5. Bake for 20–22 minutes or until lightly browned. Remove and let cool.

6. Enjoy with a cup of tea or a glass of almond milk!

Three-Ingredient Peanut Butter Cookies

Servings: 12 to 14
½ cup creamy peanut butter
⅛ cup pure maple syrup (you can add more
  if you like a sweeter taste)
1½ cups almond meal

1. Preheat oven to 350 degrees.

2. Combine the peanut butter and maple syrup in a medium mixing bowl and mix until creamy.

3. Slowly add the almond meal until it makes one solid dough ball.

4. Roll into 1-inch balls and place on a lightly greased baking sheet.

5. Bake for 6 minutes, then press the dough down with a fork.

6. Bake an additional 4–5 minutes or until the bottoms are golden brown.

7. Let cool before serving.

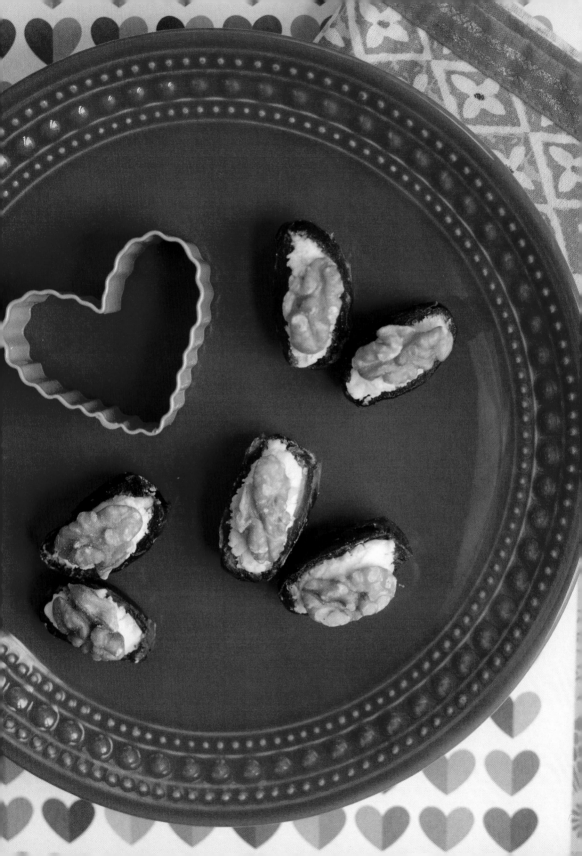

Date Night Bites

Servings: 2

- 2 dates
- 1 tablespoon goat cheese or almond butter
- 4 walnut halves

1. Cut each date in half and remove the pit.

2. Stuff each half with goat cheese or almond butter and top with a walnut half.

3. Enjoy!

OTHER STUFFING OPTIONS

Almond butter and chocolate chips

Brie, pistachio, and pomegranate

Pistachio, almond butter, and shredded coconut

Chocolate Chia Seed Pudding

Servings: 2

- 1 cup unsweetened almond or coconut milk
- 2 tablespoons raw cacao powder
- ¼ cup chia seeds
- 2 tablespoons maple syrup

1. Combine the almond or coconut milk and raw cacao powder in a small mixing bowl and mix until the cacao powder is blended in.

2. Add the chia seeds and maple syrup and mix well.

3. Chill in the fridge for 2–3 hours to set.

4. Enjoy!

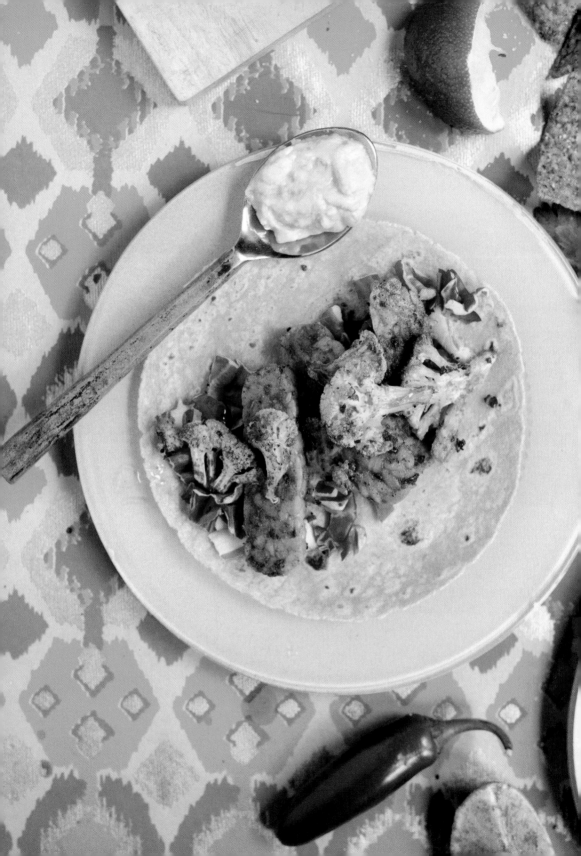

Tempeh + Cauliflower Tacos

Servings: 6

SEASONING INGREDIENTS

1 tablespoon chili powder

½ teaspoon garlic powder

¼ teaspoon onion powder

⅛ teaspoon red pepper flakes (or more to add heat!)

1 teaspoon smoked paprika

2 teaspoon cumin

2 teaspoon sea salt

½ teaspoon pepper

TACO INGREDIENTS

1 cauliflower head

1 8-ounce package of tempeh

Olive oil

1 red cabbage, chopped finely

6 tortilla shells

1. Preheat oven to 350 degrees.

2. Combine the seasoning ingredients in a small glass jar and mix thoroughly.

3. Cut the cauliflower into small pieces and place in a large bowl.

4. Cut the tempeh into strips or a small dice, whichever you prefer, and toss in the bowl with the cauliflower.

5. Drizzle the cauliflower-and-tempeh mixture with olive oil and toss until every piece is covered. Sprinkle on the taco seasoning and toss to cover.

6. Spread the mixture evenly onto a baking sheet and bake for 25–30 minutes or until your desired crispness.

7. Layer your tortilla shells with the cabbage, the cauliflower-and-tempeh mixture, and your favorite toppings!

Note: Top with your favorite toppings including guacamole, salsa, cheese, pico, etc.

PROTEIN NOTE: If you want to incorporate meat or don't have tempeh on hand, you can always substitute chicken, beef, or fish.

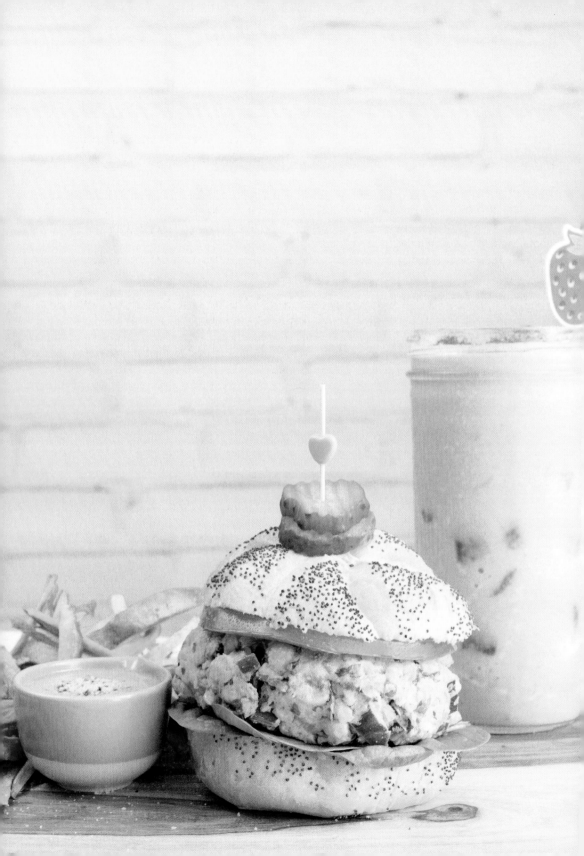

Cauliflower Burgers with Sweet Potato Fries

Servings: 4 to 6

CAULIFLOWER BURGERS

1 cauliflower head
1½ tablespoons smoked paprika, divided
2 teaspoons garlic salt, divided
½ cup millet, cooked as directed
1 15-ounce can chickpeas, drained and
    rinsed
½ cup Parmesan cheese
¼ cup chia seeds
1 tablespoon curry powder
1 garlic clove, minced
1 egg
Salt and pepper, to taste
Olive oil

1. Preheat oven to 350 degrees.

2. Cut the cauliflower head into little pieces, toss in olive oil, and place on the baking sheet. Sprinkle 1 tablespoon of smoked paprika and 1 teaspoon of garlic salt on top. Bake for 15–20 minutes.

3. In a food processor, combine millet, chickpeas, Parmesan cheese, chia seeds, curry powder, ½ tablespoon smoked paprika, 1 teaspoon garlic salt, garlic clove, egg, and most of the baked cauliflower, leaving about ¼ cup to the side.

4. Pulse in the food processor, scraping down the sides to ensure an even distribution. The patty mixture should still have some chunks of cauliflower and chickpeas in it, so don't overprocess.

5. Mix in the reserved ¼ cup of whole cauliflower into the patty mixture. Take the mix and form patties by hand.

6. In a large skillet coated with oil, pan-fry the burgers on medium-high heat for 3–4 minutes on each side or until your desired crispiness.

7. Serve with sweet potatoes fries and enjoy!

SWEET POTATO FRIES

2-4 sweet potatoes
Olive oil
Sea salt

1. Preheat oven to 350 degrees.

2. Wash and dry the sweet potatoes. Cut in half lengthwise. Continue to halve strips lengthwise to create small strips that look like fries.

3. Dip your fingers in olive oil, coat the fries, and place on a baking sheet. Sprinkle with sea salt.

4. Bake for 20 minutes or until you reach your desired crispness.

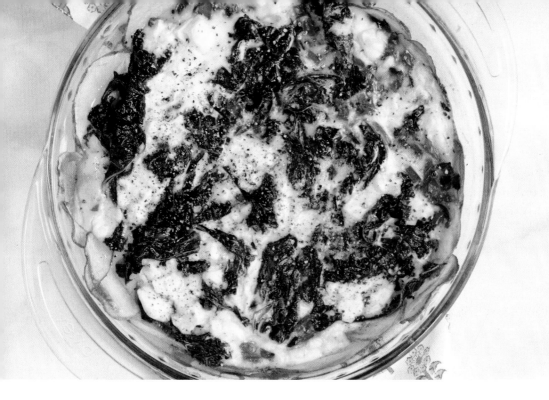

Potato Quiche

Servings: 6 to 8

1–2 potatoes, thinly sliced
1 tablespoon coconut oil
2 tablespoons olive oil
2 cloves garlic, minced
½ red onion, diced
½ red pepper, diced
1 cup kale, chopped
6 organic cage-free eggs, lightly beaten
Sea salt and pepper, to taste
Raw cheddar or feta cheese to top
   (optional)

1. Preheat oven to 400 degrees.

2. Lightly coat a pie pan with the

coconut oil and cover with the sliced potatoes. Set aside.

3. In a large skillet, heat the olive oil and add the garlic and a pinch of sea salt. Sauté for a few minutes.

4. Add the onion and red pepper and sauté until lightly browned.

5. Add the kale and sauté for 5–10 minutes, until slightly wilted.

6. Once the veggies are done, add them to the pie pan. Then add the beaten eggs and mix. Season with sea salt and pepper to taste. Top with the cheese, if desired, for an extra kick of flavor.

7. Bake for 25–30 minutes or until the eggs are fully cooked. You can test by sticking a fork in the middle: if there is no egg on the fork, you are good!

8. Enjoy!

Cinnamon Pear Salad

Servings: 6 to 8
 ½ cup walnut halves
 4-6 cups arugula
 1 pear, chopped
 3 tablespoons fresh lemon juice (1 lemon)
 3 tablespoons extra-virgin olive oil
 1 teaspoon cinnamon
 Sea salt, freshly ground black pepper, to
  taste

1. In a small dry pan over medium heat, toast the nuts, stirring frequently, until lightly toasted. Watch carefully so they don't burn. Let cool.

2. Combine the arugula and pear in a salad bowl, then add the nuts.

3. Add the lemon juice, oil, and cinnamon, and season to taste with sea salt and pepper. Stir to mix, then serve.

CREAMY

Cheese Sticks with Marinara

Servings: 6
 ⅓ cup gluten-free bread crumbs
 1 teaspoon garlic salt
 1 teaspoon onion salt
 1 tablespoon oregano or Italian herb blend
 Pinch of sea salt
 3 string cheeses
 1 egg
 Marinara sauce

1. Preheat oven to 350 degrees and set aside a parchment-lined baking sheet.

2. Combine the bread crumbs, garlic salt, onion salt, oregano, and sea salt in a small bowl and set aside.

3. Cut the string cheese in half width-wise.

4. Beat the egg in a small bowl. Dip the cheese stick in the egg and then coat it in the bread crumb mixture and place it onto the baking sheet.

5. Once all cheese sticks have been covered, sprinkle any leftover bread crumb mixture on the top.

6. Bake for 8–10 minutes or until the cheese is gooey.

7. Serve with a side of marinara sauce.

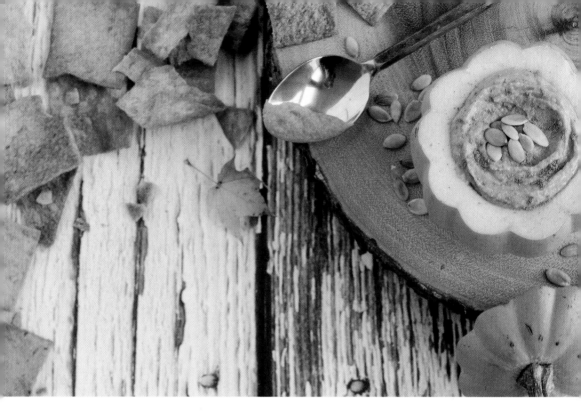

Pumpkin Pie Hummus

Servings: 4

- 1 15-ounce can chickpeas, rinsed and drained
- 7½ ounces pumpkin puree (from a 15-ounce can)
- 2 tablespoons tahini
- 4 tablespoons raw or local honey
- 1 tablespoon pumpkin pie spice
- ¼ teaspoon sea salt

1. In a blender or food processor, blend all the ingredients plus 1 tablespoon of water until smooth and creamy, pausing occasionally to scrape the inside of the bowl with a spatula. If the mixture is too thick, add another tablespoon of water.

2. Refrigerate for 2 hours in an airtight container before serving.

Note: Cinnamon sugar pita chips make this dish extra sweet!

Salsamole

Because who has time to cut vegetables when you're hangry!

Servings: 6 to 8
- 1 avocado
- 1 can of your favorite salsa
- Tortilla chips

1. De-seed and cut the avocado into cubes.

2. In a small bowl, mix the avocado and salsa.

3. Attempt to calmly enjoy the fruits of your labor. (Or stuff your face because once you guac, you can't stop.)

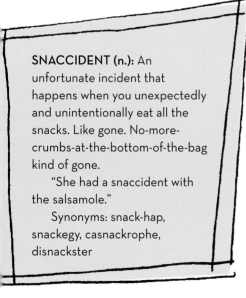

SNACCIDENT (n.): An unfortunate incident that happens when you unexpectedly and unintentionally eat all the snacks. Like gone. No-more-crumbs-at-the-bottom-of-the-bag kind of gone.

"She had a snaccident with the salsamole."

Synonyms: snack-hap, snackegy, casnackrophe, disnackster

Roasted Cauliflower Mash

Servings: 6 to 8
- 1 cauliflower head, chopped
- 1 15-ounce can chickpeas, rinsed and drained
- ½ large onion, chopped
- 3 garlic cloves
- 1-2 tablespoons olive oil
- Sea salt and ground black pepper
- 7½ ounces pumpkin puree (from a 15-ounce can)
- 2 teaspoons pumpkin pie spice
- ¼ cup almond, soy, or coconut milk
- 1 tablespoon maple syrup (optional)

1. Preheat oven to 350 degrees.

2. On a large baking sheet, place the cauliflower, chickpeas, onion, and garlic. Lightly coat with the oil. Add salt and pepper to taste. Toss with your hands until all the pieces are coated.

3. Bake for 20–25 minutes or until the cauliflower is golden brown and soft.

4. Transfer the vegetables and excess oil from the baking sheet to a high-powered blender or food processor. Add the pumpkin puree, pie spice, almond or soy or coconut milk, and maple syrup, if using. Process until it forms a smooth mash.

5. Serve immediately, or transfer the mash to a casserole dish and heat for 5–10 minutes in the oven before serving.

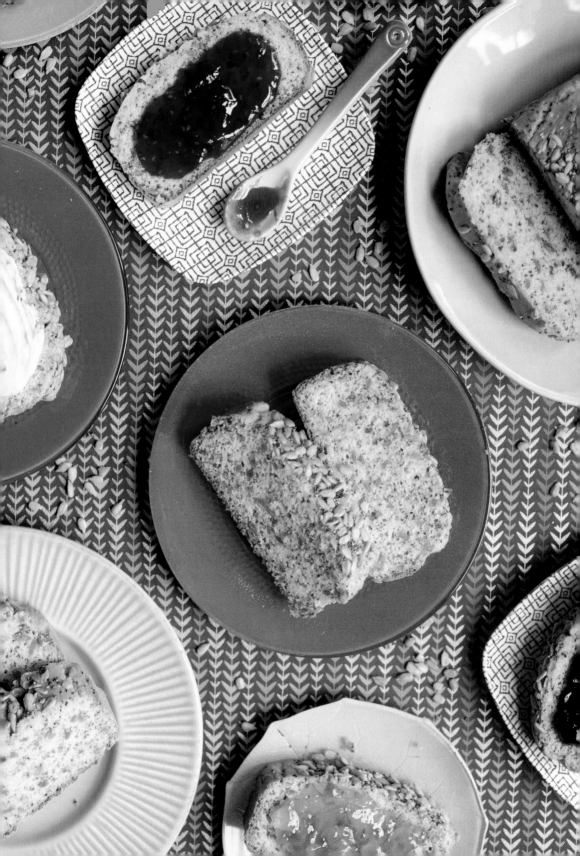

CRUNCHY

Almond Chia Bread

Servings: 8 to 10
   2 cups almond flour
   ¼ cup chia seeds
   2 teaspoons baking powder
   ½ teaspoon sea salt
   ¼ cup coconut oil
   5 eggs
   2 tablespoons maple syrup
   ½ cup sunflower seeds

1. Preheat oven to 350 degrees.

2. In a bowl or food processor, combine the almond flour, chia seeds, baking powder, and sea salt.

3. Add the coconut oil, eggs, and maple syrup, and mix or blend until smooth.

4. Add the sunflower seeds to the mixture.

5. Transfer the mixture into a parchment-lined or coconut-oil-greased loaf pan. If you have extra sunflower seeds, sprinkle them on top for an extra crunch.

6. Bake for 35–40 minutes or until the crust is golden brown.

7. Let cool for 10 minutes. Serve it sweet with some raspberry jam or savory with some avocado and sea salt.

Cucumber Cups

Servings: 16
   2 cucumbers
   8 ounces hummus
   Feta cheese

1. Cut the cucumbers in 2-inch increments.

2. Scoop out some of the seeds until the cucumber forms a little cup.

3. Fill the inside with the hummus and top with the feta cheese.

4. Enjoy!

Power Wrap

Servings: 1

 1 gluten-free tortilla (or a collard green wrap!)

 2 tablespoons hummus

 Handful of spinach

 ½ cup leftover bell peppers, carrots, cucumbers, and/or mushrooms, sliced or chopped

 1 tablespoon dried cranberries

1. Lay the tortilla flat on a clean work surface. Spread the hummus over the tortilla. Add the spinach to cover the hummus.

2. Place the veggies in the center and sprinkle with the cranberries. Roll up the tortilla and get your wrap on!

PROTEIN NOTE: For some added power, you can add grilled chicken, beef, fish, or tempeh.

Mini Veggie Muffins

Servings: 18 to 24

 2 cups quinoa or spelt flour

 Pinch of sea salt

 2 eggs, beaten

 1 cup veggies, grated or finely chopped (whatever you like/have in your refrigerator)

 ½ cup parsley, finely chopped

 1 cup soy or rice milk

1. Preheat oven to 325 degrees.

2. Mix the flour and sea salt in a bowl.

3. Make a well and add the eggs, veggies, and parsley.

4. Mix lightly, gradually adding the milk. This is supposed to be lumpy, so don't work too hard!

5. Spoon into a mini muffin tray that is lightly oiled.

6. Bake for 12–15 minutes.

7. Remove and allow to set for 10 minutes, then serve.

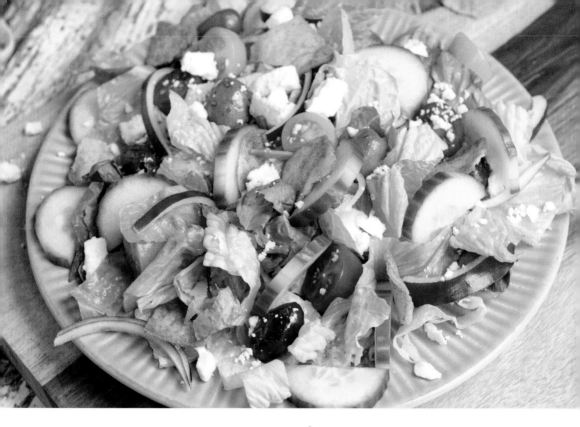

Greek Salad

Servings: 1

SALAD INGREDIENTS

2 romaine lettuce stalks, thinly sliced
6 cherry tomatoes, cut in half
¼ cucumber, cut in half circles
¼ cup crushed pita chips
Olives (optional)
Feta cheese (optional)

DRESSING INGREDIENTS

½ lemon, juiced
2 tablespoons olive oil
1 teaspoon sumac
Salt and pepper, to taste

1. Combine the salad ingredients in a medium bowl.

2. Prepare the dressing ingredients in a small bowl.

3. Add the dressing to the salad mixture, toss, and serve.

PROTEIN NOTE: Add a filet of grilled salmon, grilled shrimp, or grilled tofu or tempeh for additional protein to keep you fuller throughout the day.

DRINKS

PB + Jelly Shake

Servings: 1
- 1 frozen banana
- 4-6 strawberries
- 2 tablespoons peanut butter
- ¾ cup almond milk

Blend all the ingredients and enjoy!

Grounded and Good Smoothie

Servings: 1
- ½ pear
- ½ banana
- ½ cup almond milk
- 1 tablespoon cinnamon
- Handful of ice

Blend all the ingredients and enjoy!

No-Sheep-Counting Sleep Hack

If you are unable to fall asleep, try breathing in through your nose for three counts and out through your mouth for four counts. The repetition and the breathing will help you get to sleep in no time. No counting sheep needed.

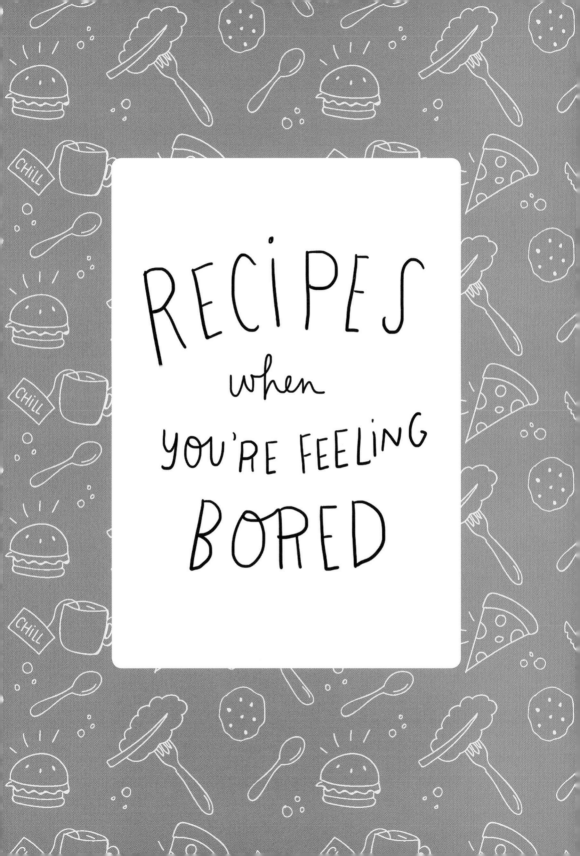

EMOTION: Bored

Did you ever have a crazy busy week and you longed for Sunday because it was the one day that you could be "lazy" and do nothing? Then Sunday rolls around and you find yourself bored out of your mind and mindlessly munching on the most random food in your house, never truly being satisfied?

Oftentimes, when we are bored, we gravitate toward food because it makes us feel accomplished. I mean, sometimes I count eating as a major accomplishment, especially when it feels like I did nothing else but waste my day. (Thanks, popcorn, for making me feel like a real winner today!)

Bored eating can also be a symptom of procrastination or feeling uninspired, especially for people who are used to being productive and motivated to create or finish things.

In this section, you will find recipes that help inspire you as well as lifestyle tips for things to do when you're bored.

SIGNS AND SYMPTOMS OF BORED EATING

- You aren't really hungry but find yourself saying, "Treat yo' self."
- You procrastinate about everything on your to-do list and eventually say "Oh yeah, I should probably eat" to distract yourself even more.
- You put off every possible item on your to-do list and replace each with a cookie.
- Even three-day-old leftovers look good.

WHAT'S (REALLY) HAPPENING TO YOUR BODY?

When you're bored, your neurotransmitters such as dopamine are also bored. So when you grab something to eat, what you are really trying to do is wake up your neurotransmitters to give you some energy, excitement, or motivation.

Food also evokes a certain level of happiness. Food can bring us joy and pleasure. So when we're bored, we feel that eating a bag of chips or a candy bar will somehow give us that happiness factor that we were looking for or provide us with some excitement in our day.

I can remember certain days when the most exciting thing that happened was eating a really good brownie from the new bakery down the street or making a delicious scone that tasted just like pizza.

When it comes to combating eating out of boredom, it's really important to ensure that you eat foods that can help

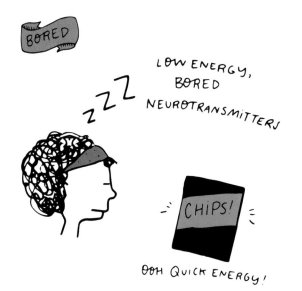

you feel motivated and centered rather than lethargic and uninspired. Also, use the act of cooking as a means to inspire you and lift you from your boredom and enhance your creativity.

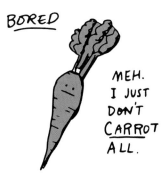

BEST FOODS KNOWN TO FIGHT OFF BOREDOM

Apples
Chickpeas
Clementines
Corn
Cucumbers
Dates
Eggplant
Jicama
Pecans
Pickles
Pumpkin seeds
Salmon
Seaweed
Spinach
Tomatoes
Zucchini

Why These Foods?

When you're bored, it's important to fuel your body with foods that will leave you feeling inspired, motivated, and ready to take action on anything but eating more food.

Omega-3s: These fatty acids help build brain cell membranes and promote new brain cell function, which can help keep your memory sharp and your creative juices flowing.

Iron: If you are feeling bored, unmotivated, or even weak, you could be low in iron. Iron deficiency can make you feel lethargic, bored, and uninspired to do anything.

OTHER TYPES OF FOODS TO EAT

Healthy Fats: Eating foods that can help increase your brain function, such as those with healthy fats, is a great way to ease out of brain fog and get you thinking and moving again.

Calming Foods: When you are procrastinating, oftentimes it's because you are so filled up with things to do that you shut down and want to do nothing. By incorporating grounding and calming foods into your diet, you can feel centered around projects instead of overwhelmed.

LIFESTYLE "FOODS"

- Make something! Have an arts and crafts bucket around so that when you get bored, you can make something fun. Maybe even make some of the household/self-care products on page 114.
- Paint your nails. Choose a color that goes with your mood!
- Unsubscribe to emails that are no longer serving you. This will help clear your space and allow new and fun things to come your way.
- Send a friend a handwritten note. Since handwritten notes are a dying breed, a little note to say "Hi!" can liven your day and a friend's day as well.
- Listen to a podcast or watch a tutorial to engage your brain and learn something new.

Chocolate Almond Tartlets

Servings: 4

CRUST INGREDIENTS

¾ cup raw almonds
12-15 dates, pitted
¼ cup chia seeds
½ teaspoon pure vanilla extra

FILLING INGREDIENTS

⅓ cup maple syrup
⅓ cup raw cacao
¼ cup coconut shreds
⅓ cup coconut oil
4 tablespoons almond butter

TOPPING OPTIONS

Coconut shreds
Cacao nibs
Chocolate chips

1. To make the crust, combine the raw almonds, dates, chia seeds, and vanilla extract in a food processor and blend until a dough ball forms. Separate the dough into four balls. Press evenly into each of four mini pie pans, covering the entire pan, and refrigerate while you make the filling.

2. To make the filling, combine the maple syrup, raw cacao, coconut shreds, and coconut oil. Use a small blender to ensure the mixture is creamy and smooth.

3. Gently pour just enough filling to cover the bottom of the crusts, and use a spoon to spread onto the sides, reserving the rest of the prepared filling. Refrigerate the filled pie pans for 10–15 minutes or until the chocolate hardens

4. Add a tablespoon of almond butter to each of the mini pies and spread evenly. Top with the remaining filling and sprinkle with toppings.

5. Refrigerate for 30 minutes before serving.

Nut Butter Fudge

Servings: 12

½ cup almond, peanut, or sunflower butter
2 tablespoons maple syrup
3 tablespoons coconut oil

1. Combine all the ingredients in a small blender and blend until smooth.

2. Pour into candy molds or spread into a small flat glass dish.

3. Freeze for 15 minutes and enjoy!

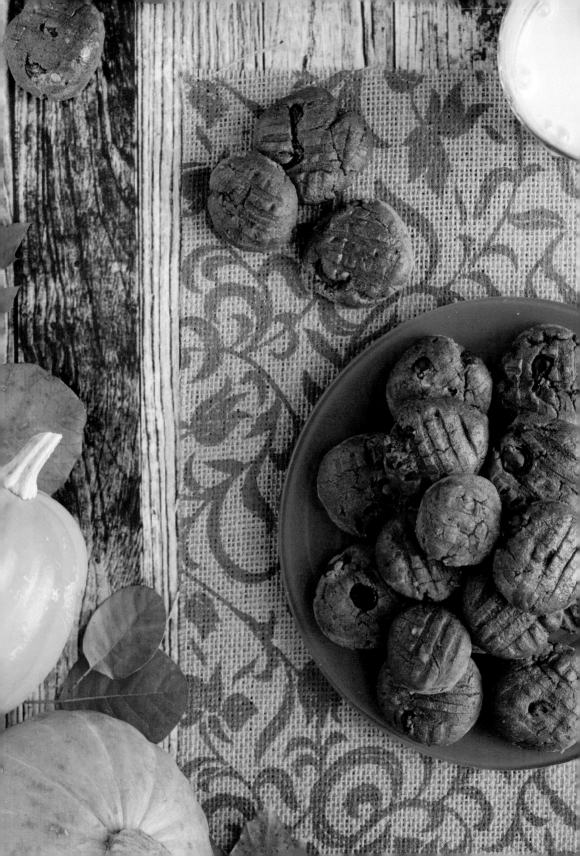

Pumpkin Spice Cookies

Servings: 22 to 25
- ½ cup pumpkin puree
- ⅓ cup maple syrup
- ¼ cup coconut oil, melted
- ½ tablespoon pure vanilla extract
- 1 cup flour (I use gluten-free cup for cup)
- ½ teaspoon baking soda
- ½ teaspoon baking powder
- Pinch of salt
- 1½ tablespoons pumpkin pie spice
- Chocolate chips (optional)

1. Preheat oven to 350 degrees.

2. In a large bowl, combine the pumpkin puree, maple syrup, coconut oil, and vanilla, and mix well.

3. In a small bowl, combine the flour, baking soda, baking powder, salt, and pumpkin pie spice.

4. Slowly add the dry mixture to the wet mixture. Use a hand mixer if needed.

5. Fold in chocolate chips, if desired.

6. Roll into 1-inch balls, place on a parchment-lined baking sheet, and press down on each ball with a fork until flat.

7. Bake for about 10 minutes.

Mini Carrot Cake Muffins

Servings: 18 to 24
- ⅓ cup coconut oil, melted
- ⅓ cup applesauce
- ⅓ cup maple syrup
- 2 eggs
- ½ tablespoon cinnamon
- ½ tablespoon pure vanilla extract
- 1 teaspoon baking soda
- ½ teaspoon baking powder
- Pinch of sea salt
- ½ cup grated carrots (approximately 6–8 large carrots)
- 1¼ cup almond flour

1. Preheat oven to 350 degrees.

2. In a large bowl, combine the coconut oil, applesauce, maple syrup, eggs, cinnamon, vanilla, baking soda, baking powder, and sea salt. Mix thoroughly.

3. Add the grated carrots and mix thoroughly.

4. Slowly add the almond flour.

5. Lightly grease mini muffin tins or use paper baking cups, and add your batter.

6. Bake for 12–15 minutes or until golden brown.

Note: Grating carrots counts as arm exercise. Who says you need weights?

Egg + Potato Tacos

Servings: 2
  1 potato, peeled and cubed small
  Olive oil
  Sea salt, to taste
  Pepper, to taste
  3 eggs
  ½ tablespoon butter
  ¼ cup black beans, drained and rinsed
  2 tortilla shells

1. Preheat oven to 350 degrees.

2. Place the cubed potatoes in a small bowl, drizzle with olive oil and sprinkle with sea salt, and toss. Transfer the potatoes to a baking sheet and bake for 15–20 minutes or until your desired crispiness.

3. Whisk the eggs and season with salt and pepper.

4. In a medium skillet, heat the butter on medium heat and add the eggs. With a wooden spoon or spatula, scramble the eggs by continuously moving them in the pan as they are heating. Once they are done, remove from the pan and set aside.

5. Heat the black beans in the same pan for a few minutes.

6. Add the eggs back into the pan, turn off the heat, and cover.

7. Remove the potatoes from the oven and add to the black-bean-and-egg mixture. Stir thoroughly.

8. Layer your tortilla shells with the egg-and-potato mixture, and top them with your favorite ingredients. Salsa, pico, or hot sauce really give the dish a nice kick of flavor.

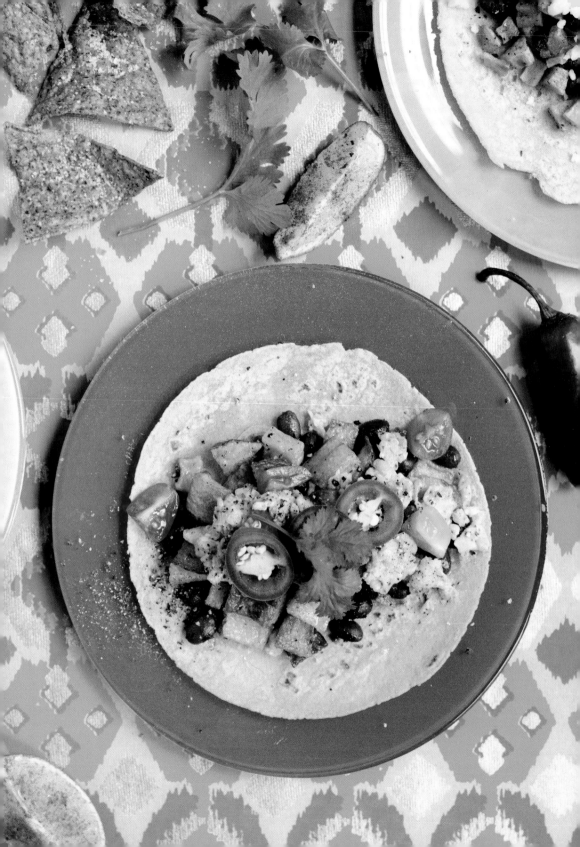

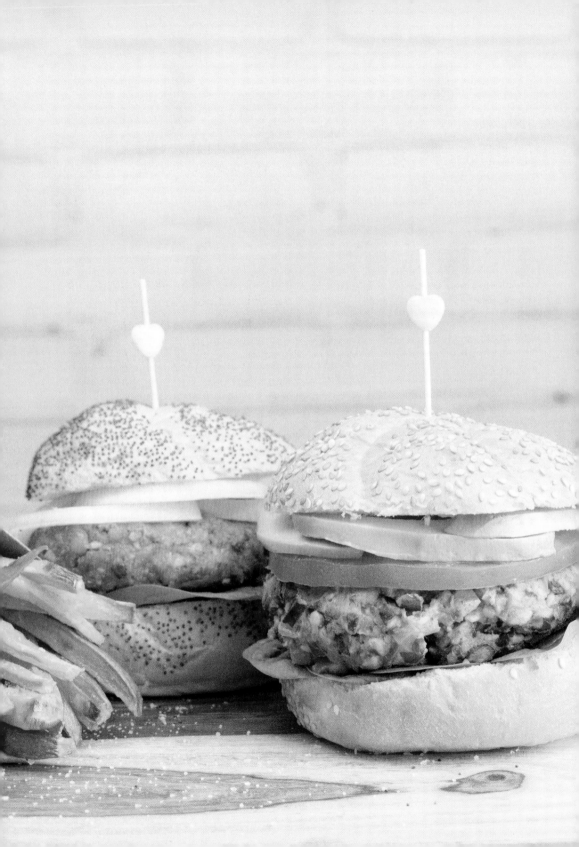

Falafel Burger

Servings: 4 to 6
- 1 15-ounce can chickpeas, rinsed and drained
- 2 tablespoons tahini
- 2 tablespoons gluten-free flour (or almond meal)
- 2 garlic cloves, minced
- 1 small red onion, diced
- 1 bunch parsley, chopped finely
- 1 teaspoon ground coriander
- 1 teaspoon cumin
- 1 teaspoon garlic salt
- ½ teaspoon onion powder
- Salt and pepper, to taste
- Olive oil

1. In a large food processor, combine all ingredients and blend gently until it forms a chunky batter, scraping down the sides as needed. Don't overprocess as it will turn to paste and you want to still be able to see the red onion and some chickpeas.

2. Take the mix and form patties by hand.

3. In a large skillet coated with oil, pan-fry the burgers on medium-high heat for 3–4 minutes on each side or until your desired crispiness.

4. Serve on a bed of greens, on a bun, or eat as is with your favorite toppings!

Za'atar Fries

Servings: 4 to 6
- 2-4 sweet potatoes
- 1-2 tablespoons za'atar seasoning
- Sea salt
- Olive oil

1. Preheat oven to 350 degrees.

2. Wash and dry the sweet potatoes. Cut in half lengthwise. From there cut small strips lengthwise. Take those strips and cut one more time down the middle. The goal is to create small strips that look like fries.

3. Dip your fingers in olive oil, coat the fries, and place on a baking sheet. Sprinkle with the za'atar seasoning and sea salt.

4. Bake for 20 minutes or until you reach your desired crispness.

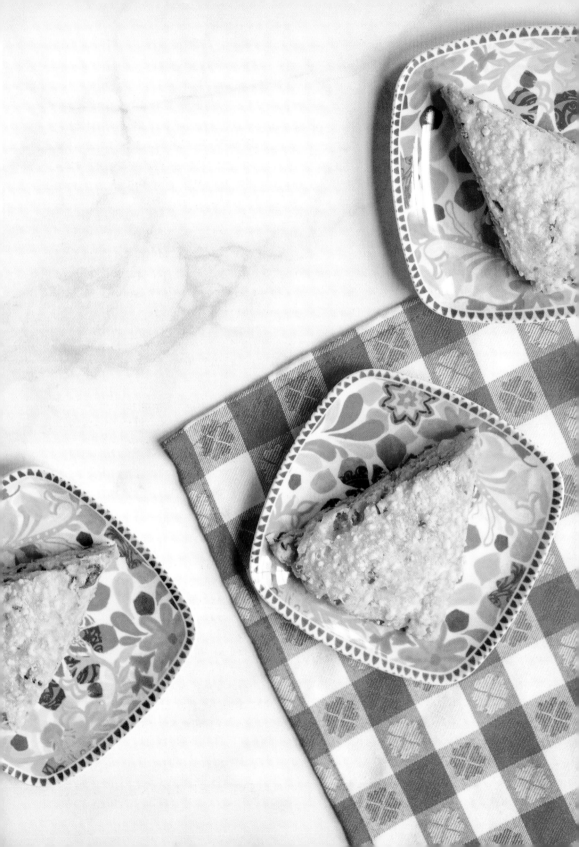

Savory Scones

Pizza Scones

Servings: 8

  2 cups gluten-free or whole grain flour, sifted
  1 tablespoon baking powder
  1 tablespoon garlic powder
  ¼ heaping teaspoon sea salt
  ½ cup cold butter, cut into pieces
  ¾ cup Asiago cheese, finely grated, divided
  ½ cup sun-dried tomatoes, grated
  10 basil leaves, chopped
  2 large eggs, divided
  ½ cup + 3 tablespoons full-fat Greek yogurt

1. Preheat oven to 450 degrees.

2. In a large bowl, mix together the flour, baking powder, garlic powder, and salt. Add the pieces of butter, working them in to form even crumbs.

3. Add ½ cup of the cheese, the sun-dried tomatoes, and basil.

4. Beat together 1 egg and 1 egg yolk. Reserve the extra egg white. Add the yogurt and whisk together.

5. Slowly pour the wet ingredients into the dry ingredients until a dough ball is formed. You may need to mix with your hands to form the ball.

6. Lightly sprinkle flour on a parchment-lined baking sheet. Press the dough into a ½-inch-thick circle. Cut into 8 slices, just as you would a pizza.

7. Place the scones about an inch or two apart on the baking sheet. Whisk the reserved egg white until foamy, and brush on the tops of the scones. Sprinkle with remaining Asiago cheese.

8. Bake for 10–12 minutes or until they're golden brown. Remove, cool, and serve!

PROTEIN NOTE: If you eat meat and don't have sun-dried tomatoes on hand, you can always substitute pepperoni.

Cheddar and Jalapeño Scones

Servings: 8

  2 cups gluten-free or whole grain flour, sifted
  1 tablespoon baking powder
  1 tablespoon garlic powder
  ¼ heaping teaspoon sea salt
  ½ cup cold butter, cut into pieces
  ¾ cup fresh cheddar cheese, grated or
    chopped, divided
  2 jalapeños, finely chopped
  2 large eggs, divided
  ½ cup + 2 tablespoons full-fat Greek yogurt

1. Preheat oven to 450 degrees.

2. In a large bowl, mix together the flour, baking powder, garlic powder, and salt. Add the pieces of butter, working them in to form even crumbs.

3. Add ½ cup of the cheese and the jalapeños.

4. Beat together 1 egg and 1 egg yolk. Reserve the extra egg white. Add the yogurt and whisk together.

5. Slowly pour the wet ingredients into the dry ingredients until a dough ball is formed. You may need to mix with your hands to form the ball.

6. Lightly sprinkle flour on a parchment-lined baking sheet. Press the dough into a ½-inch-thick circle. Cut into 8 slices, just as you would a pizza.

7. Place the scones about an inch or two apart on the baking sheet. Whisk the reserved egg white until foamy, and brush on the tops of the scones. Sprinkle with remaining cheddar cheese.

8. Bake for 10–12 minutes or until they're golden brown. Remove, cool, and serve!

Zucchini "Pasta"

Servings: 4
  2 small/medium zucchinis
  Olive oil
  1 small yellow onion, diced
  3 garlic cloves, minced
  1 26-ounce jar marinara sauce
  Parmesan cheese
  Basil

1. Use a spiralizer to make zoodles (zucchini + noodles = zoodles).

2. In a large skillet, warm olive oil on medium heat and toss in the onion, sautéing for about 5–6 minutes.

3. Add the garlic and toss for about 1 minute or until fragrant.

4. Add the zoodles and toss for about 5 minutes or until coated and lightly cooked. Be careful not to overcook them as they will get mushy.

5. Add the desired amount of marinara sauce and mix until warm.

6. Serve topped with cheese and basil.

PROTEIN NOTE: Add cooked ground beef to your marinara if you want a meatier "pasta."

Pineapple Peanut Noodles

Servings: 4

SAUCE

1½ tablespoons olive oil
½ tablespoon sesame oil
4 garlic cloves, minced
1½ tablespoons liquid amino acids, soy
 sauce, or tamari sauce
1 tablespoon rice wine vinegar
2 teaspoons grated ginger
1 cup peanut butter
1 20-ounce can diced pineapple (no sugar
 added), divided
2 tablespoons chili paste

NOODLES AND VEGGIES

1 8-ounce package buckwheat noodles
 (soba or linguine will work, too!)
Snow peas
Radishes
Red peppers
Cucumbers
Carrots

GARNISH OPTIONS

Chopped peanuts
Chopped cilantro
Chopped scallions
Chopped jalapeños
Lime juice
Sesame seeds

1. In a medium saucepan on low heat, combine the olive oil, sesame oil, and garlic. Heat for 2–3 minutes or until fragrant.

2. Add the liquid amino acids, rice wine vinegar, ginger, peanut butter, pineapple juice from the can, and chili paste.

3. Blend the pineapple itself in a blender until smooth, and add to the sauce. Stir until everything is thoroughly mixed. Let simmer on low for 10–15 minutes, stirring occasionally.

4. Prepare the noodles as directed.

5. Prep as many veggies as you'd like. Julienne them or finely chop.

6. Rinse the noodles in cold water, and stir in the sauce and veggies until evenly coated. Serve immediately or let chill for 30 minutes.

7. Top with peanuts, cilantro, scallions, jalapeños, lime juice, sesame seeds, and/or other garnishes you like.

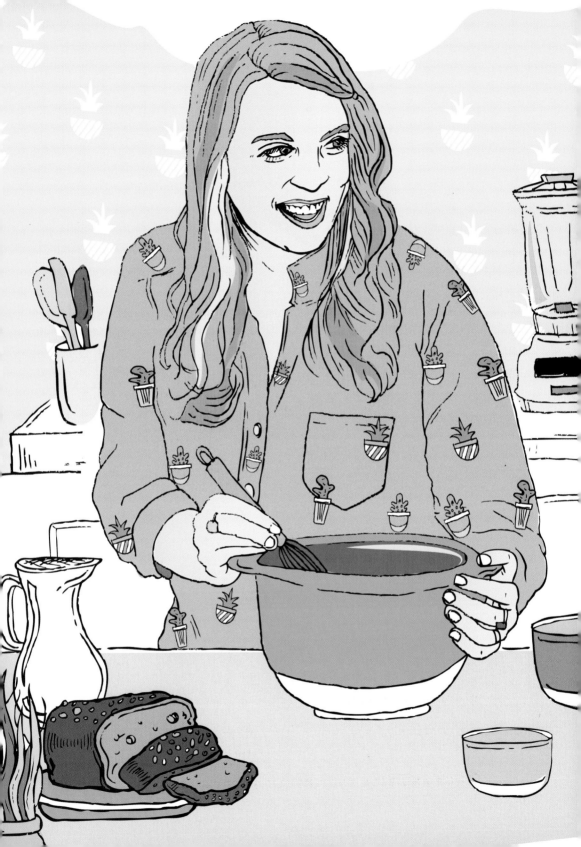

Creamy Sweet Potato Soup

Servings: 4

1 small yellow onion, diced
Olive oil
2 garlic cloves, minced
1 large sweet potato, peeled and diced
1 tablespoon yellow curry powder
¼ teaspoon red pepper flakes
Dash of cayenne pepper
1 13.5-ounce can coconut milk
Salt and pepper, to taste
Hemp seeds

1. In a medium-large skillet over medium heat, sauté the onion in olive oil for about 5 minutes or until tender.

2. Add the garlic and sauté for about 1 minute or until fragrant.

3. Add the sweet potato and toss for about 10 minutes.

4. Add the curry powder, red pepper flakes, cayenne, coconut milk, salt, and pepper. Mix thoroughly and let simmer on low for about 15 minutes, stirring occasionally.

5. Once the sweet potatoes are tender, transfer the mixture to a large blender and blend until smooth and creamy.

6. Serve and top with the hemp seeds!

Almond Flour Drop Biscuits

Servings: 8 to 12

2 cups almond flour
¼ teaspoon baking soda
¼ teaspoon baking powder
Pinch of sea salt
¼ cup coconut oil, melted
2 eggs
2 tablespoons maple syrup
½ teaspoon apple cider vinegar

1. Preheat oven to 350 degrees.

2. In a large bowl, combine the dry ingredients.

3. Add the liquid ingredients and mix thoroughly until a dough ball forms.

4. On a parchment-lined baking sheet, drop ice-cream-scoop-size balls of dough about 2 inches apart.

5. Bake 15–17 minutes or until lightly browned.

Open-Faced Veggie Pot Pie

Servings: 4

2 potatoes, peeled and cubed
1 small yellow onion, diced
2 carrots, diced small
Olive oil
4 garlic cloves, minced
8 ounces oyster or shiitake mushrooms, chopped small
1 bay leaf
1 teaspoon granulated garlic
2-3 tablespoons flour (I use gluten-free cup for cup)
2 cups vegetable stock
1 cup frozen peas
Salt and pepper, to taste
Paprika

1. Soak your potatoes in a bowl of water.

2. In a medium pot, cook the onion and carrots in olive oil over medium heat for 5–6 minutes or until the onion is translucent.

3. Add the minced garlic, mushrooms, bay leaf, and granulated garlic, and cook for about 10 minutes on medium heat, tossing throughout.

4. Drain the water from the potatoes.

5. Add the flour to the sautéing vegetables and mix until dissolved.

6. Add the potatoes and cook for 4–5 minutes.

7. Add the vegetable stock, mix thoroughly, and let simmer for 15 minutes, stirring occasionally.

8. Add the peas and cook an additional 10–15 minutes or until the potatoes are cooked through. Remove the bay leaf.

9. Serve with Almond Flour Drop Biscuits and sprinkle with paprika.

PROTEIN NOTE: Add cooked chicken if you want a Chicken Pot Pie instead.

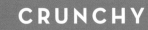

CRUNCHY

Crispy Chickpeas

Servings: 2
  1 tablespoon olive oil
  1 15-ounce can of chickpeas, drained and
    dried
  Sea salt and pepper, to taste

1. Preheat oven to 350 degrees.

2. Take a baking sheet and lightly coat with the olive oil.

3. Roll the chickpeas around in the oil until they are lightly coated.

4. Salt and pepper the chickpeas to your taste.

5. Bake for about 25 minutes or until the chickpeas are lightly browned and crunchy.

FLAVOR ADAPTATIONS

Depending on your mood, try some of these fun flavor options:

  Rosemary
  Dill
  Cinnamon sugar

Cinnamon Apple Crunch

It's like Cinnamon Toast Crunch . . . except not. For those times when you want something crunchy and satisfying with little to no effort. So in that regard, I guess, it is like Cinnamon Toast Crunch.

Servings: 8
  1 apple
  ½ to 1 tablespoon peanut or almond butter
  Handful of walnuts
  Ground cinnamon, to taste

1. Slice your apple.

2. Add a little peanut or almond butter to each slice, top with walnuts, and sprinkle with desired cinnamon.

3. Enjoy with a glass of your favorite milk. Or don't. That's cool, too.

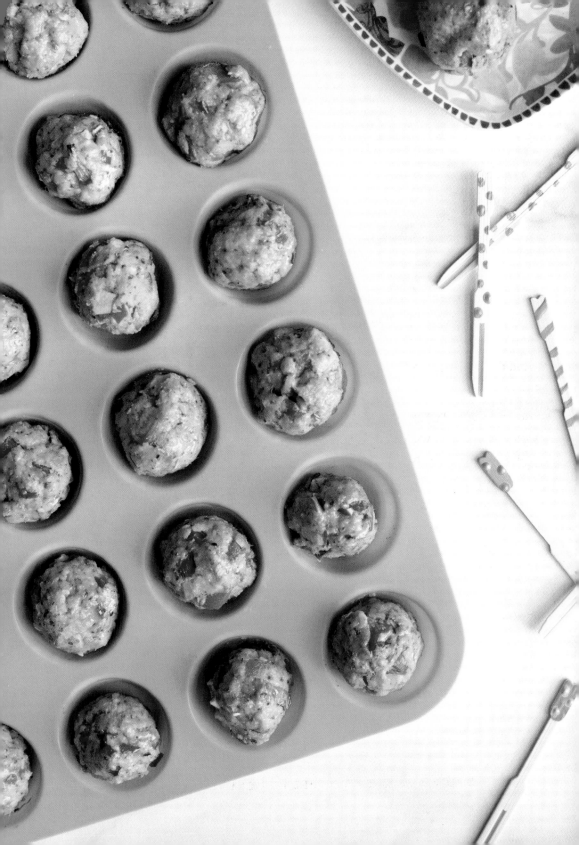

Za'atar Salmon Bites

Servings: 18 to 24
2 6-ounce cans salmon, deboned
½ red onion, diced
½ red pepper, diced
½ cup almond flour
1 tablespoon za'atar
Salt and pepper, to taste
2 eggs

1. Drain the water from the canned salmon and place the salmon in a medium bowl.

2. Add the red onion and red pepper to the bowl.

3. Add the almond flour, za'atar, salt, and pepper to the bowl. Mix with your hands until the spices are nice and even throughout.

4. Add the two eggs and mix with your hands until the dough starts to form a ball.

5. Make small balls and place them in a greased or lined mini muffin pan or use a silicone muffin mold.

Rosemary Cheese Crackers

Servings: 25 to 30
1 cup almond meal
1 cup Parmesan cheese
2 tablespoons rosemary
Pinch of salt
½ teaspoon baking soda
1 egg
1 tablespoon olive oil

1. Preheat oven to 350 degrees.

2. In a large bowl or food processor, combine the almond meal, Parmesan cheese, rosemary, salt, and baking soda.

3. Add the egg and olive oil and mix until well combined. Use your hands to form a large ball of dough.

4. Take a teaspoon-size piece of dough and roll into a ball. Gently press down to make a circle and place it on a parchment-lined baking sheet. Continue until all the dough is gone.

5. Bake for 12–14 minutes or until the crackers are light brown on the bottom.

Zucchini Pizza Bites

Servings: 10 to 12
  1 zucchini
  Pizza sauce
  Mozzarella cheese

1. Cut the zucchini into ½-inch rounds.

2. Top with the sauce and cheese.

3. You can eat them raw or hot. If you want them hot, bake at 350 degrees for 10–15 minutes.

4. Eat. Them. All.

PROTEIN NOTE: If you want some additional meat flavor, you can chop up pepperoni and add to the pizza bites.

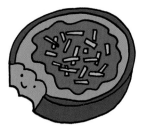

Strawberry Milkshake

Servings: 1
  1 frozen banana
  ½ cup strawberries
  ½ cup almond milk

Blend all ingredients and enjoy!

Vegan Egg Nog

Servings: 1
  1 banana
  2 dates, pitted
  1 teaspoon cinnamon
  1 cup almond milk

Blend all the ingredients and enjoy!

Green Boredom Smoothie

Servings: 1
  1 cup spinach
  1 kale stalk, de-stemmed
  ½ cup frozen berries
  1 tablespoon almond butter
  1 teaspoon spirulina powder
  1 cup nut milk

Blend all the ingredients and enjoy!

GRATITUDE

Eric: Thanks for being the most supportive and funny agent a girl can ask for. You believed in my idea, championed me along the way, and answered way too many texts.

Laura: From the very first moment we met, you believed in the book and me. So excited to have had your insight and support in order to create and write the best book possible. Also, we are the only author-editor duo who I know to have weathered a storm for vegan ice cream.

Amanda: Thank you for encouraging me to pursue this book traditionally. If it wasn't for your late-night pep talk, I'm pretty sure this book wouldn't even exist. You are the best!

Quelcy: Thank you for putting life and style to my recipes and my life. So glad to have your creative and humorous lens on this project to make it that much better. Also, dogs.

Kate: The second I saw your nineties music reference on one of the book illustrations, I knew it was meant to be. Thanks so much for your love of food puns and truly making my quirkiness come to life visually.

Sarah: Thank you for the many photo shoots, dance sessions, and your amazing ability to always capture exactly who I am.

Derek: My love. Thank you for your ongoing support and culinary tips and tricks. Also, thanks for being the best taste-tester and not settling until each recipe was perfected.

Creative Council: Hey, remember that time I invited you all to come and hear my silly jokes and crazy ideas? Thanks for helping me refine my book and make it what it is today!

Team Rocks: I couldn't have asked for a better group of agent siblings. Thanks for all the help, pep talks, and jokes you have provided me! You all rock!

INDEX

INDEX

INDEX

INDEX